Virtual Clinical Excursions—General Hospital

for

Williams:
Fundamental Concepts and Skills for Nursing,
Fifth Edition

CCalna
56dtJQYxhJKW

Virtual Clinical Excursions—General Hospital

for

Williams:
Fundamental Concepts and Skills for Nursing,
Fifth Edition

prepared by

Jennifer A. Morris, RN, BSN
Assistant Professor of Vocational Nursing
South Plains College
Levelland, Texas

software developed by

Wolfsong Informatics, LLC
Tucson, Arizona

ELSEVIER

ELSEVIER

3251 Riverport Lane
Maryland Heights, Missouri 63043

VIRTUAL CLINICAL EXCURSIONS—GENERAL HOSPITAL FOR
WILLIAMS: FUNDAMENTAL CONCEPTS AND SKILLS FOR NURSING,
FIFTH EDITION

ISBN: 978-0-323-42962-7

Notice

Knowledge and best practice in this field are constantly changing. As new research and experience broaden our understanding, changes in research methods, professional practices, or medical treatment may become necessary.

Practitioners and researchers must always rely on their own experience and knowledge in evaluating and using any information, methods, compounds, or experiments described herein. In using such information or methods they should be mindful of their own safety and the safety of others, including parties for whom they have a professional responsibility.

With respect to any drug or pharmaceutical products identified, readers are advised to check the most current information provided (i) on procedures featured or (ii) by the manufacturer of each product to be administered, to verify the recommended dose or formula, the method and duration of administration, and contraindications. It is the responsibility of practitioners, relying on their own experience and knowledge of their patients, to make diagnoses, to determine dosages and the best treatment for each individual patient, and to take all appropriate safety precautions.

To the fullest extent of the law, neither the Publisher nor the authors, contributors, or editors, assume any liability for any injury and/or damage to persons or property as a matter of products liability, negligence or otherwise, or from any use or operation of any methods, products, instructions, or ideas contained in the material herein.

ISBN: 978-0-323-42962-7

Printed in the United States of America

Last digit is the print number: 9 8 7 6 5 4 3 2 1

Workbook
prepared by

Jennifer A. Morris, RN, BSN
Assistant Professor of Vocational Nursing
South Plains College
Levelland, Texas

Textbook

Patricia O'Neill, MSN, RN, CCRN
Nursing Instructor
DeAnza College
Cupertino, California

Table of Contents
Virtual Clinical Excursions Workbook

Getting Set Up with VCE Online 1

A Quick Tour 3

A Detailed Tour 19

Reducing Medication Errors 31

Lesson 1   Priority Setting and Goal Development (Chapters 2, 4, 5, and 26) 37

Lesson 2   Critical Thinking and Problem Solving (Chapters 4, 5, and 28) 43

Lesson 3   Communication and the Nurse-Patient Relationship (Chapters 7 and 8) 51

Lesson 4   Documentation of Nursing Care (Chapter 7) 61

Lesson 5   Patient Teaching (Chapter 9) 69

Lesson 6   Nursing Care of the Older Adult: Common Physical Care Issues
            (Chapters 13, 18, 40, and 41) 77

Lesson 7   Nursing Care of the Older Adult: Psychosocial Care
            (Chapters 11, 13, and 41) 85

Lesson 8   Loss, Grief, and the Dying Patient (Chapters 14 and 15) 93

Lesson 9   Pain, Comfort, and Sleep (Chapters 14, 31, and 32) 101

Lesson 10   Activity, Mobility, and Skin Care (Chapters 17, 18, 19, 38, and 39) 111

Lesson 11   Vital Signs, Health Status Assessment, and Data Collection
            (Chapters 5, 21, and 22) 119

Lesson 12   Diagnostic Testing and Specimen Collection (Chapter 24) 129

Lesson 13   Nutrition, Fluid, and Electrolytes (Chapters 25, 26, and 27) 135

Lesson 14   Promoting Respiration and Oxygenation (Chapters 25 and 28) 143

Lesson 15   Promoting Urinary and Bowel Elimination (Chapters 29 and 30) 151

Lesson 16   Preparation for Drug Administration (Chapters 33 and 34) 159

Lesson 17   Oral Medication Administration (Chapters 33 and 34) 167

Lesson 18   Administering Injections and Topical Medications (Chapters 34 and 35) 175

Lesson 19   Caring for Patients Receiving Intravenous Therapy (Chapter 36) 181

Lesson 20   Care of the Surgical Patient: Pre- and Intraoperative Care (Chapter 37) 189

Lesson 21   Care of the Surgical Patient: Postoperative Care
            (Chapters 27, 37, 38, and 39) 197

Table of Contents
Williams:
Fundamental Concepts and Skills for Nursing, Fifth Edition

Unit I: Introduction to Nursing and the Health Care System

1 Nursing and the Health Care System
2 Concepts of Health, Illness, Stress, and Health Promotion (Lesson 1)
3 Legal and Ethical Aspects of Nursing

Unit II: The Nursing Process

4 The Nursing Process and Critical Thinking (Lessons 1 and 2)
5 Assessment, Nursing Diagnosis, and Planning (Lessons 1, 2, and 11)
6 Implementation and Evaluation

Unit III: Communication in Nursing

7 Documentation of Nursing Care (Lessons 3 and 4)
8 Communication and the Nurse-Patient Relationship (Lesson 3)
9 Patient Education and Health Promotion (Lesson 5)
10 Delegation, Leadership, and Management

Unit IV: Developmental, Psychosocial, and Cultural Considerations

11 Growth and Development: Infancy Through Adolescence (Lesson 7)
12 Adulthood and the Family
13 Promoting Healthy Adaptation to Aging (Lessons 6 and 7)
14 Cultural and Spiritual Aspects of Patient Care (Lessons 8 and 9)
15 Loss, Grief, and End-of-Life Care (Lesson 8)

Unit V: Basic Nursing Skills

16 Infection Prevention and Control: Protective Mechanisms and Asepsis
17 Infection Prevention and Control in the Hospital and Home (Lesson 10)
18 Safe Lifting, Moving, and Positioning of Patients (Lessons 6 and 10)
19 Assisting with Hygiene, Personal Care, Skin Care, and the Prevention of Pressure Ulcers (Lesson 10)
20 Patient Environment and Safety
21 Measuring Vital Signs (Lesson 11)
22 Assessing Health Status (Lesson 11)
23 Admitting, Transferring, and Discharging Patients
24 Diagnostic Tests and Specimen Collection (Lesson 12)

Unit VI: Meeting Basic Physiologic Needs

25 Fluid, Electrolyte, and Acid-Base Balance (Lessons 13 and 14)
26 Concepts of Basic Nutrition and Cultural Considerations (Lessons 1 and 13)
27 Nutritional Therapy and Assisted Feeding (Lessons 13 and 21)
28 Assisting with Respiration and Oxygen Delivery (Lessons 2 and 14)
29 Promoting Urinary Elimination (Lesson 15)
30 Promoting Bowel Elimination (Lesson 15)
31 Pain, Comfort, and Sleep (Lesson 9)
32 Complementary and Alternative Therapies (Lesson 9)

Unit VII: Medication Administration

33 Pharmacology and Preparation for Drug Administration (Lessons 16 and 17)
34 Administering Oral, Topical, and Inhalant Medications (Lessons 16, 17, and 18)
35 Administering Intradermal, Subcutaneous, and Intramuscular Injections (Lesson 18)
36 Administering Intravenous Solutions and Medications (Lesson 19)

Unit VIII: Care of the Surgical and Immobile Patient

37 Care of the Surgical Patient (Lessons 20 and 21)
38 Providing Wound Care and Treating Pressure Ulcers (Lessons 10 and 21)
39 Promoting Musculoskeletal Function (Lessons 10 and 21)

Unit IX: Caring for the Elderly

40 Common Physical Care Problems of the Older Adult (Lesson 6)
41 Common Psychosocial Care Problems of Older Adults (Lessons 6 and 7)

Appendixes

Appendix A Standard Steps for All Nursing Procedures

Appendix B NFLPN Nursing Practice Standards for the Licensed Practical/Vocational Nurse

Appendix C ANA Code of Ethics

Appendix D Standard Precautions

Appendix E Common Laboratory Test Values

Appendix F NANDA-I Approved Nursing Diagnoses, 2015-2017

Reader References

Glossary

GETTING SET UP WITH VCE ONLINE ───────────

The product you have purchased is part of the Evolve Learning System. Please read the following information thoroughly to get started.

■ HOW TO ACCESS YOUR VCE RESOURCES ON EVOLVE

There are two ways to access your VCE Resources on Evolve:

1. If your instructor has enrolled you in your VCE Evolve Resources, you will receive an email with your registration details.

2. If your instructor has asked you to self-enroll in your VCE Evolve Resources, he or she will provide you with your Course ID (for example, 1479_jdoe73_0001). You will then need to follow the instructions at https://evolve.elsevier.com/cs/studentEnroll.html.

■ HOW TO ACCESS THE ONLINE VIRTUAL HOSPITAL

The online virtual hospital is available through the Evolve VCE Resources. There is no software to download or install: the online virtual hospital runs within your Internet browser, using a pop-up window.

■ TECHNICAL REQUIREMENTS

- Broadband connection (DSL or cable)
- 1024 x 768 screen resolution
- Mozilla Firefox 18.0, Internet Explorer 9.0, Google Chrome, or Safari 5 (or higher)
  Note: Pop-up blocking software/settings must be disabled.
- Adobe Acrobat Reader
- Additional technical requirements available at http://evolvesupport.elsevier.com

■ HOW TO ACCESS THE WORKBOOK

There are two ways to access the workbook portion of *Virtual Clinical Excursions:*

1. Print workbook
2. An electronic version of the workbook, available within the VCE Evolve Resources

■ TECHNICAL SUPPORT

Technical support for *Virtual Clinical Excursions* is available by visiting the Technical Support Center at http://evolvesupport.elsevier.com or by calling 1-800-222-9570 inside the United States and Canada.

Trademarks: Windows® and Macintosh® are registered trademarks.

A QUICK TOUR

Welcome to *Virtual Clinical Excursions—General Hospital*, a virtual hospital setting in which you can work with multiple complex patient simulations and also learn to access and evaluate the information resources that are essential for high-quality patient care. The virtual hospital, Pacific View Regional Hospital, has realistic architecture and access to patient rooms, a Nurses' Station, and a Medication Room.

■ BEFORE YOU START

Make sure you have your textbook nearby when you use *Virtual Clinical Excursions*. You will want to consult topic areas in your textbook frequently while working with the virtual hospital and workbook.

■ HOW TO SIGN IN

- Enter your name in the first section of the sign-in window.
- Next, specify the floor on which you will work by clicking the corresponding button under **Select Floor**. For this quick tour, choose **Medical-Surgical**.
- Now choose one of the four periods of care in which to work. In Periods of Care 1 through 3, you can actively engage in patient assessment, entry of data in the electronic patient record (EPR), and medication administration. Period of Care 4 presents the day in review. Click the appropriate button under **Select Period of Care**. (For this quick tour, choose **Period of Care 1: 0730-0815**.)
- This takes you to the Patient List screen (see the *How to Select a Patient* section below). Only the patients on the Medical-Surgical Floor are available. Note that the virtual time is provided in the box at the lower left corner of the screen (0730, because we chose Period of Care 1).

Note: If you choose to work during Period of Care 4: 1900-2000, the Patient List screen is skipped because you are not able to visit patients or administer medications during the shift. Instead, you are taken directly to the Nurses' Station, where the records of all the patients on the floor are available for your review.

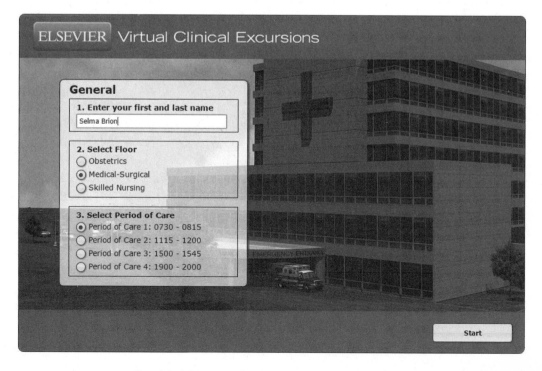

■ PATIENT LIST

MEDICAL-SURGICAL UNIT

Harry George (Room 401)
Osteomyelitis—A 54-year-old Caucasian male admitted from a homeless shelter with an infected leg. He has complications of type 2 diabetes mellitus, alcohol abuse, nicotine addiction, poor pain control, and complex psychosocial issues.

Jacquline Catanazaro (Room 402)
Asthma—A 45-year-old Caucasian female admitted with an acute asthma exacerbation and suspected pneumonia. She has complications of chronic schizophrenia, noncompliance with medication therapy, obesity, and herniated disc.

Piya Jordan (Room 403)
Bowel obstruction—A 68-year-old Asian female admitted with a colon mass and suspected adenocarcinoma. She undergoes a right hemicolectomy. This patient's complications include atrial fibrillation, hypokalemia, and symptoms of meperidine toxicity.

Clarence Hughes (Room 404)
Degenerative joint disease—A 73-year-old African-American male admitted for a left total knee replacement. His preparations for discharge are complicated by the development of a pulmonary embolus and the need for ongoing intravenous therapy.

Pablo Rodriguez (Room 405)
Metastatic lung carcinoma—A 71-year-old Hispanic male admitted with symptoms of dehydration and malnutrition. He has chronic pain secondary to multiple subcutaneous skin nodules and psychosocial concerns related to family issues with his approaching death.

Patricia Newman (Room 406)
Pneumonia—A 61-year-old Caucasian female admitted with worsening pulmonary function and an acute respiratory infection. Her chronic emphysema is complicated by heavy smoking, hypertension, and malnutrition. She needs access to community resources such as a smoking cessation program and meal assistance.

SKILLED NURSING UNIT

William Jefferson (Room 501)
Alzheimer's disease—A 75-year-old African-American male admitted for stabilization of type 2 diabetes and hypertension following a recent acute care admission for a urinary tract infection and sepsis. His complications include episodes of acute delirium and a history of osteoarthritis.

Kathryn Doyle (Room 503)
Rehabilitation post left hip replacement—A 79-year-old Caucasian female admitted following a complicated recovery from an ORIF. She is experiencing symptoms of malnutrition and depression due to unstable family dynamics, placing her at risk for elder abuse.

Goro Oishi (Room 505)
Hospice care—A 66-year-old Asian male admitted following an acute care admission for an intracerebral hemorrhage and resulting coma. Family-staff interactions provide opportunities to explore death and dying issues related to conflict about advanced life support and cultural and religious differences.

OBSTETRICS UNIT

Dorothy Grant (Room 201)
30-week intrauterine pregnancy—A 25-year-old Caucasian female multipara admitted with abdominal trauma following a domestic violence incident. Her complications include preterm labor and extensive social issues such as acquiring safe housing for her family upon discharge.

■ HOW TO SELECT A PATIENT

- You can choose one or more patients to work with from the Patient List by checking the box to the left of the patient name(s). For this quick tour, select Piya Jordan and Pablo Rodriguez. (In order to receive a scorecard for a patient, the patient must be selected before proceeding to the Nurses' Station.)
- Click on **Get Report** to the right of the medical records number (MRN) to view a summary of the patient's care during the 12-hour period before your arrival on the unit.
- After reviewing the report, click on **Go to Nurses' Station** in the right lower corner to begin your care. (*Note:* If you have been assigned to care for multiple patients, you can click on **Return to Patient List** to select and review the report for each additional patient before going to the Nurses' Station.)

Note: Even though the Patient List is initially skipped when you sign in to work for Period of Care 4, you can still access this screen if you wish to review the shift report for any of the patients. To do so, simply click on **Patient List** near the top left corner of the Nurses' Station (or click on the clipboard to the left of the Kardex). Then click on **Get Report** for the patient(s) whose care you are reviewing. This may be done during any period of care.

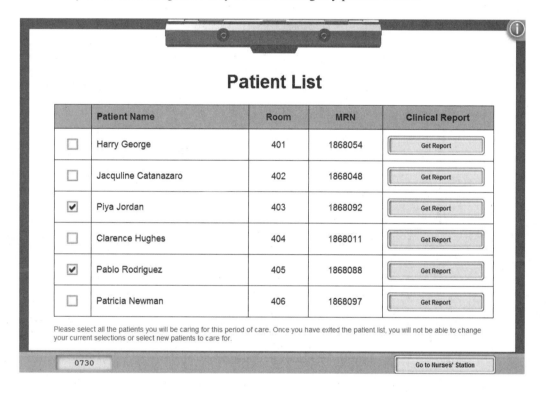

■ HOW TO FIND A PATIENT'S RECORDS

NURSES' STATION

Within the Nurses' Station, you will see:

1. A clipboard that contains the patient list for that floor.
2. A chart rack with patient charts labeled by room number, a notebook labeled Kardex, and a notebook labeled MAR (Medication Administration Record).
3. A desktop computer with access to the Electronic Patient Record (EPR).
4. A tool bar across the top of the screen that can also be used to access the Patient List, EPR, Chart, MAR, and Kardex. This tool bar is also accessible from each patient's room.
5. A Drug Guide containing information about the medications you are able to administer to your patients.
6. A Laboratory Guide containing normal value ranges for all laboratory tests you may come across in the virtual patient hospital.
7. A tool bar across the bottom of the screen that can be used to access the Floor Map, patient rooms, Medication Room, and Drug Guide.

As you run your cursor over an item, it will be highlighted. To select, simply click on the item. As you use these resources, you will always be able to return to the Nurses' Station by clicking on the **Return to Nurses' Station** bar located in the right lower corner of your screen.

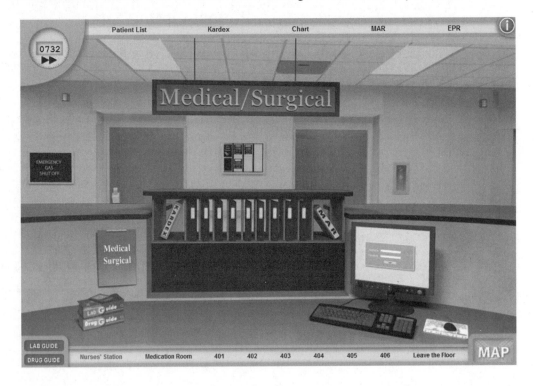

MEDICATION ADMINISTRATION RECORD (MAR)

The MAR icon located on the tool bar at the top of your screen accesses current 24-hour medications for each patient. Click on the icon and the MAR will open. (*Note:* You can also access the MAR by clicking on the MAR notebook on the far right side of the book rack in the center of the screen.) Within the MAR, tabs on the right side of the screen allow you to select patients by room number. Be careful to make sure you select the correct tab number for *your* patient rather than simply reading the first record that appears after the MAR opens. Each MAR sheet lists the following:

- Medications
- Route and dosage of each medication
- Times of administration of each medication

Note: The MAR changes each day. Expired MARs are stored in the patients' charts.

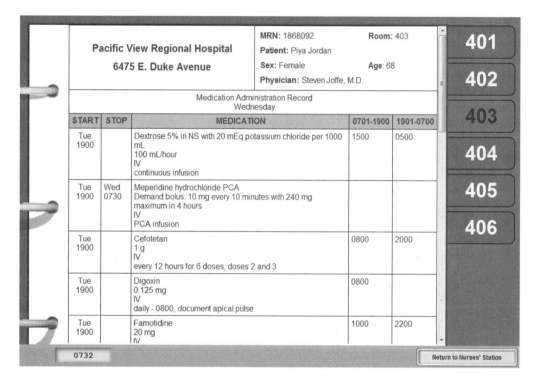

		Pacific View Regional Hospital	6475 E. Duke Avenue		
		MRN: 1868092		Room: 403	
		Patient: Piya Jordan			
		Sex: Female		Age: 68	
		Physician: Steven Joffe, M.D.			

Medication Administration Record
Wednesday

START	STOP	MEDICATION	0701-1900	1901-0700
Tue 1900		Dextrose 5% in NS with 20 mEq potassium chloride per 1000 mL 100 mL/hour IV continuous infusion	1500	0500
Tue 1900	Wed 0730	Meperidine hydrochloride PCA Demand bolus: 10 mg every 10 minutes with 240 mg maximum in 4 hours IV PCA infusion		
Tue 1900		Cefotetan 1 g IV every 12 hours for 6 doses, doses 2 and 3	0800	2000
Tue 1900		Digoxin 0.125 mg IV daily - 0800, document apical pulse	0800	
Tue 1900		Famotidine 20 mg IV	1000	2200

0732

Return to Nurses' Station

401
402
403
404
405
406

CHARTS

To access patient charts, either click on the **Chart** icon at the top of your screen or anywhere within the chart rack in the center of the Nurses' Station screen. When the close-up view appears, the individual charts are labeled by room number. To open a chart, click on the room number of the patient whose chart you wish to review. The patient's name and allergies will appear on the left side of the screen, along with a list of tabs on the right side of the screen, allowing you to view the following data:

- Allergies
- Physician's Orders
- Physician's Notes
- Nurse's Notes
- Laboratory Reports
- Diagnostic Reports
- Surgical Reports
- Consultations

- Patient Education
- History and Physical
- Nursing Admission
- Expired MARs
- Consents
- Mental Health
- Admissions
- Emergency Department

Information appears in real time. The entries are in reverse chronologic order, so use the down arrow at the right side of each chart page to scroll down to view previous entries. Flip from tab to tab to view multiple data fields or click on **Return to Nurses' Station** in the lower right corner of the screen to exit the chart.

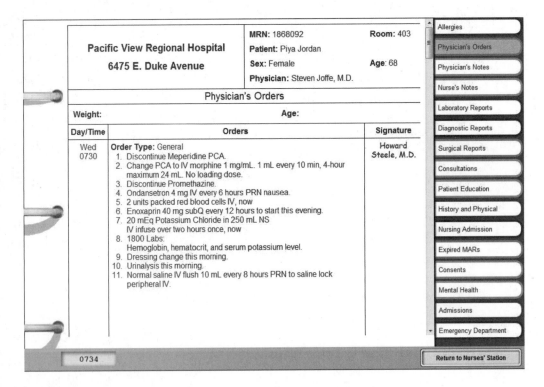

ELECTRONIC PATIENT RECORD (EPR)

The EPR can be accessed from the computer in the Nurses' Station or from the EPR icon located in the tool bar at the top of your screen. To access a patient's EPR:
- Click on either the computer screen or the **EPR** icon.
- Your username and password are automatically filled in.
- Click on **Login** to enter the EPR.
- *Note:* Like the MAR, the EPR is arranged numerically. Thus when you enter, you are initially shown the records of the patient in the lowest room number on the floor. To view the correct data for *your* patient, remember to select the correct room number, using the drop-down menu for the Patient field at the top left corner of the screen.

The EPR used in Pacific View Regional Hospital represents a composite of commercial versions being used in hospitals. You can access the EPR:
- to review existing data for a patient (by room number).
- to enter data you collect while working with a patient.

The EPR is updated daily, so no matter what day or part of a shift you are working, there will be a current EPR with the patient's data from the past days of the current hospital stay. This type of simulated EPR allows you to examine how data for different attributes have changed over time, as well as to examine data for all of a patient's attributes at a particular time. The EPR is fully functional (as it is in a real-life hospital). You can enter such data as blood pressure, breath sounds, and certain treatments. The EPR will not, however, allow you to enter data for a previous time period. Use the arrows at the bottom of the screen to move forward and backward in time.

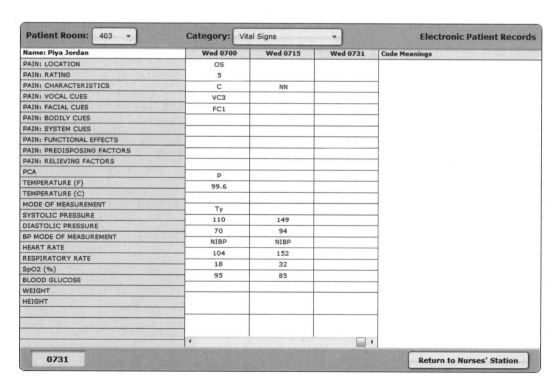

Patient Room: 403	Category: Vital Signs			Electronic Patient Records
Name: Piya Jordan	**Wed 0700**	**Wed 0715**	**Wed 0731**	**Code Meanings**
PAIN: LOCATION	OS			
PAIN: RATING	5			
PAIN: CHARACTERISTICS	C	NN		
PAIN: VOCAL CUES	VC3			
PAIN: FACIAL CUES	FC1			
PAIN: BODILY CUES				
PAIN: SYSTEM CUES				
PAIN: FUNCTIONAL EFFECTS				
PAIN: PREDISPOSING FACTORS				
PAIN: RELIEVING FACTORS				
PCA	P			
TEMPERATURE (F)	99.6			
TEMPERATURE (C)				
MODE OF MEASUREMENT	Ty			
SYSTOLIC PRESSURE	110	149		
DIASTOLIC PRESSURE	70	94		
BP MODE OF MEASUREMENT	NIBP	NIBP		
HEART RATE	104	152		
RESPIRATORY RATE	18	32		
SpO2 (%)	95	85		
BLOOD GLUCOSE				
WEIGHT				
HEIGHT				

0731   Return to Nurses' Station

At the top of the EPR screen, you can choose patients by their room numbers. In addition, you have access to 17 different categories of patient data. To change patients or data categories, click the down arrow to the right of the room number or category.

The categories of patient data in the EPR are as follows:

- Vital Signs
- Respiratory
- Cardiovascular
- Neurologic
- Gastrointestinal
- Excretory
- Musculoskeletal
- Integumentary
- Reproductive
- Psychosocial
- Wounds and Drains
- Activity
- Hygiene and Comfort
- Safety
- Nutrition
- IV
- Intake and Output

Remember, each hospital selects its own codes. The codes used in the EPR at Pacific View Regional Hospital may be different from ones you have seen in your clinical rotations. Take some time to acquaint yourself with the codes. Within the Vital Signs category, click on any item in the left column (e.g., Pain: Characteristics). In the far-right column, you will see a list of code meanings for the possible findings and/or descriptors for that assessment area.

You will use the codes to record the data you collect as you work with patients. Click on the box in the last time column to the right of any item and wait for the code meanings applicable to that entry to appear. Select the appropriate code to describe your assessment findings and type it in the box. (*Note:* If no cursor appears within the box, click on the box again until the blue shading disappears and the blinking cursor appears.) Once the data are typed in this box, they are entered into the patient's record for this period of care only.

To leave the EPR, click on **Exit EPR** in the bottom right corner of the screen.

■ VISITING A PATIENT

From the Nurses' Station, click on the room number of the patient you wish to visit (in the tool bar at the bottom of your screen). Once you are inside the room, you will see a still photo of your patient in the top left corner. To verify that this is the correct patient, click on the **Check Armband** icon to the right of the photo. The patient's identification data will appear. If you click on **Check Allergies** (the next icon to the right), a list of the patient's allergies (if any) will replace the photo.

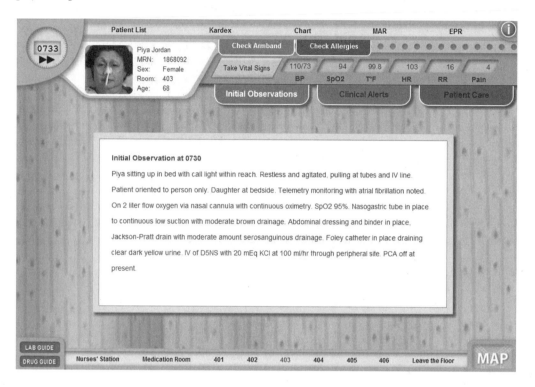

Also located in the patient's room are multiple icons you can use to assess the patient or the patient's medications. A virtual clock is provided in the upper left corner of the room to monitor your progress in real time. (*Note:* The fast-forward icon within the virtual clock will advance the time by 2-minute intervals when clicked.)

- The tool bar across the top of the screen allows you to check the **Patient List**, access the **EPR** to check or enter data, and view the patient's **Chart**, **MAR**, or **Kardex**.

- The **Take Vital Signs** icon allows you to measure the patient's up-to-the-minute blood pressure, oxygen saturation, temperature, heart rate, respiratory rate, and pain level.

- Each time you enter a patient's room, you are given an Initial Observation report to review (in the text box under the patient's photo). These notes are provided to give you a "look" at the patient as if you had just stepped into the room. You can also click on the **Initial Observations** icon to return to this box from other views within the patient's room. To the right of this icon is **Clinical Alerts**, a resource that allows you to make decisions about priority medication interventions based on emerging data collected in real time. Check this screen throughout your period of care to avoid missing critical information related to recently ordered or STAT medications.

- Clicking on **Patient Care** opens up three specific learning environments within the patient room: **Physical Assessment**, **Nurse-Client Interactions**, and **Medication Administration**.

- To perform a **Physical Assessment**, choose a body area (such as **Head & Neck**) from the column of yellow buttons. This activates a list of system subcategories for that body area (e.g., see **Sensory**, **Neurologic**, etc. in the green boxes). After you select the system you wish to evaluate, a brief description of the assessment findings will appear in a box to the right. A still photo provides a "snapshot" of how an assessment of this area might be done or what the finding might look like. For every body area, you can also click on **Equipment** on the right side of the screen.

- To the right of the Physical Assessment icon is **Nurse-Client Interactions**. Clicking on this icon will reveal the times and titles of any videos available for viewing. (*Note:* If the video you wish to see is not listed, this means you have not yet reached the correct virtual time to view that video. Check the virtual clock; you may return to access the video once its designated time has occurred—as long as you do so within the same period of care. Or you can click on the fast-forward icon within the virtual clock to advance the time by 2-minute intervals. You will then need to click again on **Patient Care** and **Nurse-Client Interactions** to refresh the screen.) To view a listed video, click on the white arrow to the right of the video title. Use the control buttons below the video to start, stop, pause, rewind, or fast-forward the action or to mute the sound.

- **Medication Administration** is the pathway that allows you to review and administer medications to a patient after you have prepared them in the Medication Room. This process is also addressed further in the *How to Prepare Medications* section below and in *Medications* in **A Detailed Tour**. For additional hands-on practice, see *Reducing Medication Errors* below **A Quick Tour** and **A Detailed Tour** in your resources.

■ HOW TO CHANGE PATIENTS, CHANGE FLOORS, OR CHANGE PERIODS OF CARE

How to Change Patients, Floors, or Periods of Care: To change patients, simply click on the new patient's room number. (You cannot receive a scorecard for a new patient, however, unless you have already selected that patient on the Patient List screen.) To change to a new period of care, to change floors, or to restart the virtual clock, click on **Leave the Floor** and then on **Restart the Program**.

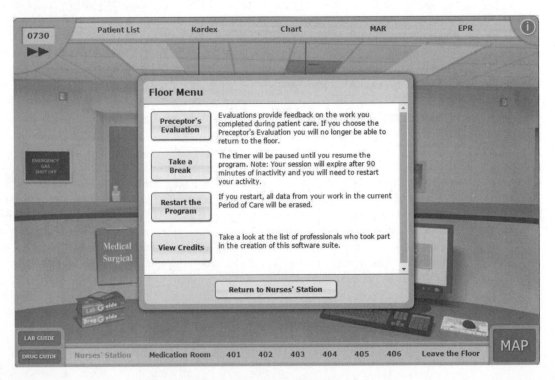

■ HOW TO PREPARE MEDICATIONS

From the Nurses' Station or the patient's room, you can access the Medication Room by clicking on the icon in the tool bar at the bottom of your screen to the left of the patient room numbers.

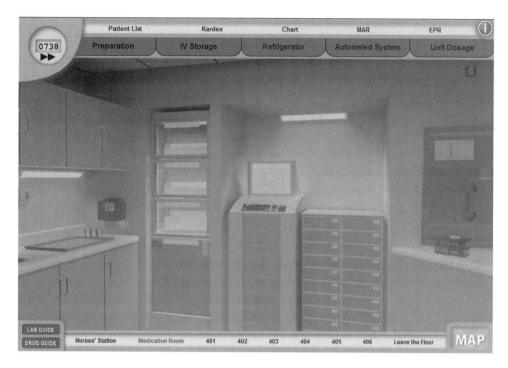

In the Medication Room you have access to the following (from left to right):

- A preparation area is located on the counter under the cabinets. To begin the medication preparation process, click on the tray on the counter or click on the **Preparation** icon at the top of the screen. The next screen leads you through a specific sequence (called the Preparation Wizard) to prepare medications one at a time for administration to a patient. However, no medication has been selected at this time. We will do this while working with a patient in **A Detailed Tour**. To exit this screen, click on **View Medication Room**.

- To the right of the cabinets (and above the refrigerator), IV storage bins are provided. Click on the bins themselves or on the **IV Storage** icon at the top of the screen. The bins are labeled **Microinfusion**, **Small Volume**, and **Large Volume**. Click on an individual bin to see a list of its contents. If you needed to prepare an IV medication at this time, you could click on the medication and its label would appear to the right under the patient's name. (*Note:* You can **Open** and **Close** any medication label by clicking the appropriate icon.) Next, you would click **Put Medication on Tray**. If you ever change your mind or decide that you have put the incorrect medication on the tray, you can reverse your actions by highlighting the medication on the tray and then clicking **Put Medication in Bin**. Click **Close Bin** in the right bottom corner to exit. **View Medication Room** brings you back to a full view of the entire room.

- A refrigerator is located under the IV storage bins to hold any medications that must be stored below room temperature. Click on the refrigerator door or on the **Refrigerator** icon at the top of the screen. Then click on the close-up view of the door to access the medications. When you are finished, click **Close Door** and then **View Medication Room**.

- To prepare controlled substances, click the **Automated System** icon at the top of the screen or click the computer monitor located to the right of the IV storage bins. A login screen will appear; your name and password are automatically filled in. Click **Login**. Select the patient for whom you wish to access medications; then select the correct medication drawer to open (they are stored alphabetically). Click **Open Drawer**, highlight the proper medication, and choose **Put Medication on Tray**. When you are finished, click **Close Drawer** and then **View Medication Room**.

- Next to the Automated System is a set of drawers identified by patient room number. To access these, click on the drawers or on the **Unit Dosage** icon at the top of the screen. This provides a close-up view of the drawers. To open a drawer, click on the room number of the patient you are working with. Next, click on the medication you would like to prepare for the patient, and a label will appear, listing the medication strength, units, and dosage per unit. To exit, click **Close Drawer**; then click **View Medication Room**.

At any time, you can learn about a medication you wish to prepare for a patient by clicking on the **Drug** icon in the bottom left corner of the medication room screen or by clicking the **Drug Guide** book on the counter to the right of the unit dosage drawers. The **Drug Guide** provides information about the medications commonly included in nursing drug handbooks. Nutritional supplements and maintenance intravenous fluid preparations are not included. Highlight a medication in the alphabetical list; relevant information about the drug will appear in the screen below. To exit, click **Return to Medication Room**.

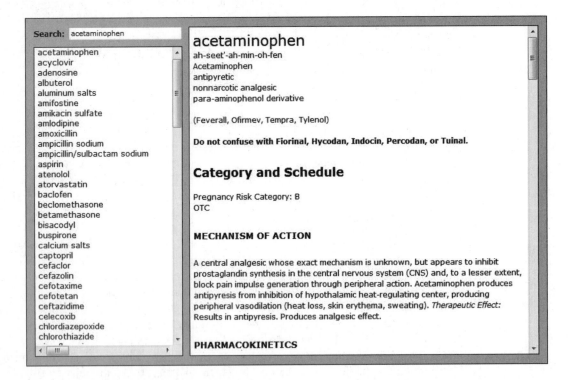

To access the MAR from the Medication Room and to review the medications ordered for a patient, click on the **MAR** icon located in the tool bar at the top of your screen and then click on the correct tab for your patient's room number. You may also click the **Review MAR** icon in the tool bar at the bottom of your screen from inside each medication storage area.

After you have chosen and prepared medications, go to the patient's room to administer them by clicking on the room number in the bottom tool bar. Inside the patient's room, click **Patient Care** and then **Medication Administration** and follow the proper administration sequence.

■ PRECEPTOR'S EVALUATIONS

When you have finished a session, click on **Leave the Floor** to go to the Floor Menu. At this point, you can click on the top icon (**Preceptor's Evaluation**) to receive a scorecard that provides feedback on the work you completed during patient care.

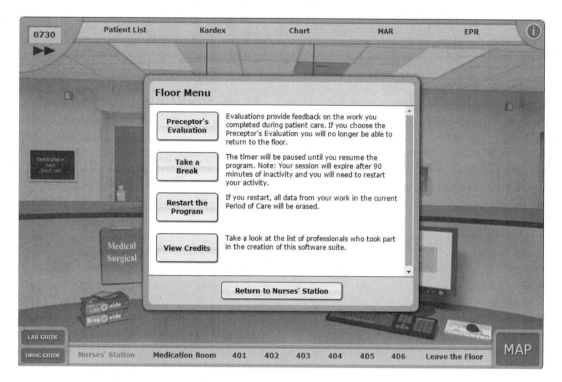

Evaluations are available for each patient you selected when you signed in for the current period of care. Click on the **Medication Scorecard** icon to see an example.

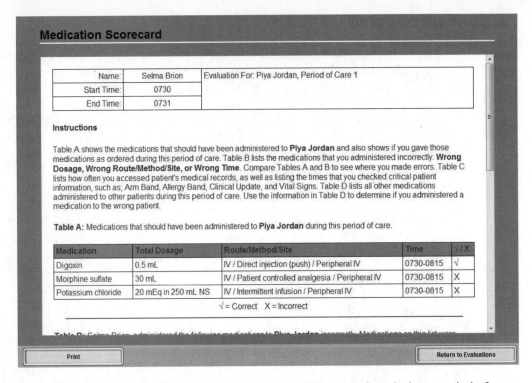

The scorecard compares the medications you administered to a patient during a period of care with what should have been administered. Table A lists the correct medications. Table B lists any medications that were administered incorrectly.

Remember, not every medication listed on the MAR should necessarily be given. For example, a patient might have an allergy to a drug that was ordered, or a medication might have been improperly transcribed to the MAR. Predetermined medication "errors" embedded within the program challenge you to exercise critical thinking skills and professional judgment when deciding to administer a medication, just as you would in a real hospital. Use all your available resources, such as the patient's chart and the MAR, to make your decision.

Table C lists the resources that were available to assist you in medication administration. It also documents whether and when you accessed these resources. For example, did you check the patient armband or perform a check of vital signs? If so, when?

You can click **Print** to get a copy of this report if needed. When you have finished reviewing the scorecard, click **Return to Evaluations** and then **Return to Menu**.

■ FLOOR MAP

To get a general sense of your location within the hospital, you can click on the **Map** icon found in the lower right corner of most of the screens in the *Virtual Clinical Excursions—General Hospital* program. (*Note:* If you are following this quick tour step by step, you will need to **Restart the Program** from the Floor Menu, sign in again, and go to the Nurses' Station to access the map.) When you click the **Map** icon, a floor map appears, showing the layout of the floor you are currently on, as well as a directory of the patients and services on that floor. As you move your cursor over the directory list, the location of each room is highlighted on the map (and vice versa). The floor map can be accessed from the Nurses' Station, Medication Room, and each patient's room.

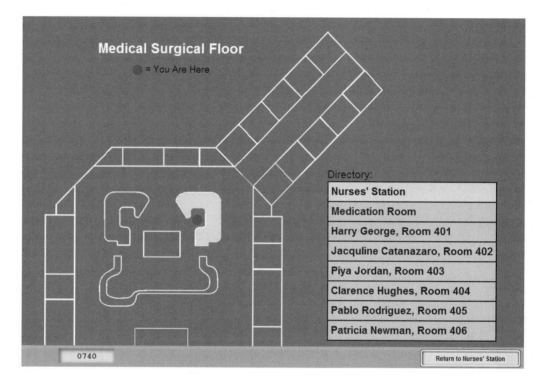

A DETAILED TOUR

If you wish to more thoroughly understand the capabilities of *Virtual Clinical Excursions—General Hospital*, take a detailed tour by completing the following section. During this tour, we will work with a specific patient to introduce you to all the different components and learning opportunities available within the software.

■ WORKING WITH A PATIENT

Sign in for Period of Care 1 (0730-0815). From the Patient List, select Piya Jordan and Pablo Rodriguez; however, do not go to the Nurses' Station yet.

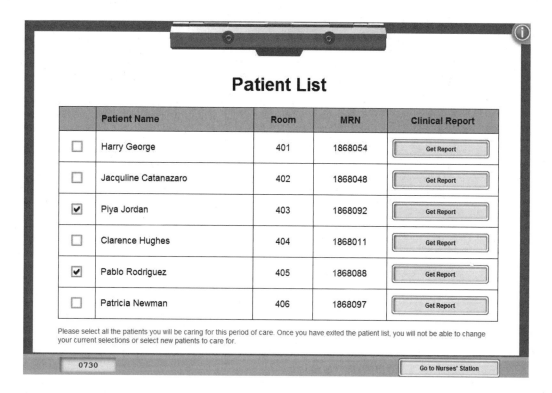

■ REPORT

In hospitals, when one shift ends and another begins, the outgoing nurse who attended a patient will give a verbal and sometimes a written summary of that patient's condition to the incoming nurse who will assume care for the patient. This summary is called a report and is an important source of data to provide an overview of a patient. Your first task is to get the clinical report on Piya Jordan. To do this, click **Get Report** in the far right column in this patient's row. From a brief review of this summary, identify the problems and areas of concern that you will need to address for this patient.

When you have finished noting any areas of concern, click **Go to Nurses' Station**.

■ CHARTS

You can access Piya Jordan's chart from the Nurses' Station or from the patient's room (403). From the Nurses' Station, click on the chart rack or on the **Chart** icon in the tool bar at the top of your screen. Next, click on the chart labeled **403** to open the medical record for Piya Jordan. Click on the **Emergency Department** tab to view a record of why this patient was admitted.

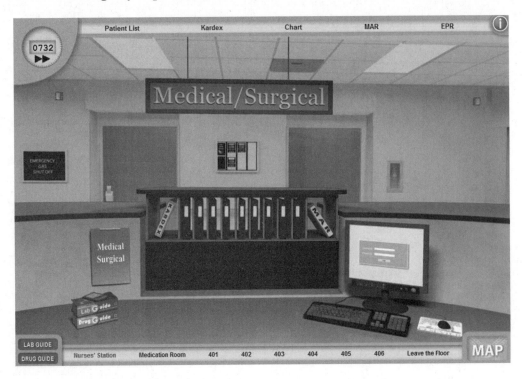

How many days has Piya Jordan been in the hospital?

What tests were done upon her arrival in the Emergency Department and why?

What was her reason for admission?

You should also click on **Diagnostic Reports** to learn what additional tests or procedures were performed and when. Finally, review the **Nursing Admission** and **History and Physical** to learn about the health history of this patient. When you are done reviewing the chart, click **Return to Nurses' Station**.

■ MEDICATIONS

Open the Medication Administration Record (MAR) by clicking on the **MAR** icon in the tool bar at the top of your screen. *Remember:* The MAR automatically opens to the first occupied room number on the floor—which is not necessarily your patient's room number! Because you need to access Piya Jordan's MAR, click on tab **403** (her room number). Always make sure you are giving the *Right Drug to the Right Patient!*

Examine the list of medications ordered for Piya Jordan. In the table below, list the medications that need to be given during this period of care (0730-0815). For each medication, note the dosage, route, and time to be given.

Time	Medication	Dosage	Route

Click on **Return to Nurses' Station**. Next, click on **403** on the bottom tool bar and then verify that you are indeed in Piya Jordan's room. Select **Clinical Alerts** (the icon to the right of Initial Observations) to check for any emerging data that might affect your medication administration priorities. Next, go to the patient's chart (click on the **Chart** icon; then click on **403**). When the chart opens, select the **Physician's Orders** tab.

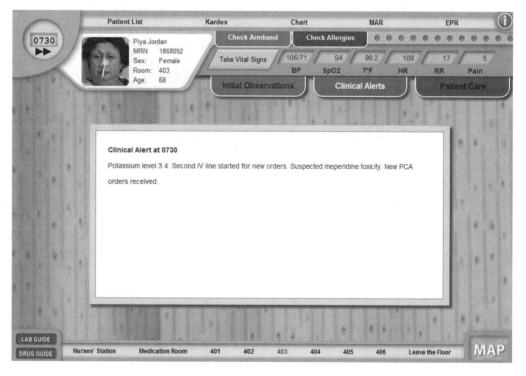

Review the orders. Have any new medications been ordered? Return to the MAR (click **Return to Room 403**; then click **MAR**). Verify that any new medications have been correctly transcribed to the MAR. Mistakes are sometimes made in the transcription process in the hospital setting, and it is sound practice to double-check any new order.

Are there any patient assessments you will need to perform before administering these medications? If so, return to Room 403 and click on **Patient Care** and then **Physical Assessment** to complete those assessments before proceeding.

Now click on the **Medication Room** icon in the tool bar at the bottom of your screen to locate and prepare the medications for Piya Jordan.

In the Medication Room, you must access the medications for Piya Jordan from the specific dispensing system in which each medication is stored. Locate each medication that needs to be given in this time period and click on **Put Medication on Tray** as appropriate. (*Hint:* Look in **Unit Dosage** drawer first.) When you are finished, click on **Close Drawer** and then on **View Medication Room**. Now click on the medication tray on the counter on the left side of the medication room screen to begin preparing the medications you have selected. (*Remember:* You can also click **Preparation** in the tool bar at the top of the screen.)

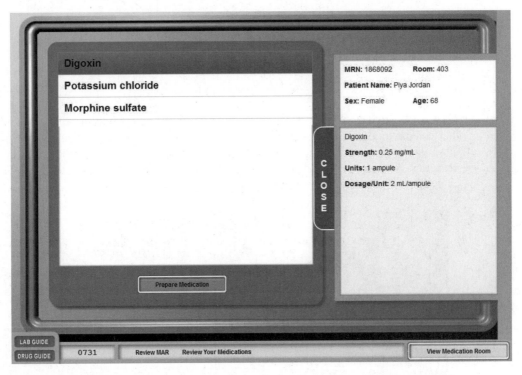

In the preparation area, you should see a list of the medications you put on the tray in the previous steps. Click on the first medication and then click **Prepare**. Follow the onscreen instructions of the Preparation Wizard, providing any data requested. As an example, let's follow the preparation process for digoxin, one of the medications due to be administered to Piya Jordan during this period of care. To begin, click to select **Digoxin**; then click **Prepare**. Now work through the Preparation Wizard sequence as detailed below:

> Amount of medication in the ampule: 2 mL.
> Enter the amount of medication you will draw up into a syringe: **0.5** mL.
> Click **Next**.
> Select the patient you wish to set aside the medication for: **Room 403, Piya Jordan**.
> Click **Finish**.
> Click **Return to Medication Room**.

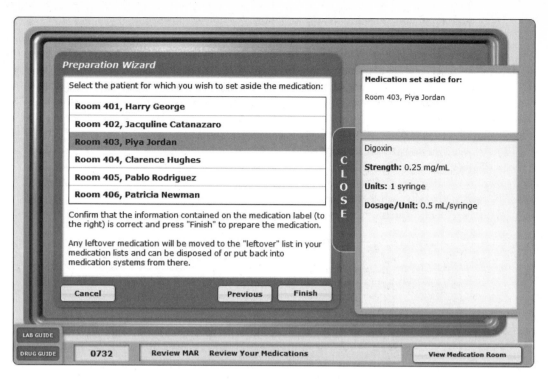

Follow this same basic process for the other medications due to be administered to Piya Jordan during this period of care. (*Hint:* Look in **IV Storage** and **Automated System**.)

PREPARATION WIZARD EXCEPTIONS

- Some medications in *Virtual Clinical Excursions—General Hospital* are preprepared by the pharmacy (e.g., IV antibiotics) and taken to the patient room as a whole. This is common practice in most hospitals.
- Blood products are not administered by students through the *Virtual Clinical Excursions—General Hospital* simulations because blood administration follows specific protocols not covered in this program.
- The *Virtual Clinical Excursions—General Hospital* simulations do not allow for mixing more than one type of medication, such as regular and Lente insulins, in the same syringe. In the clinical setting, when multiple types of insulin are ordered for a patient, the regular insulin is drawn up first, followed by the longer-acting insulin. Insulin is always administered in a special unit-marked syringe.

Now return to Room 403 (click on **403** on the bottom tool bar) to administer Piya Jordan's medications.

At any time during the medication administration process, you can perform a further review of systems, take vital signs, check information contained within the chart, or verify patient identity and allergies. Inside Piya Jordan's room, click **Take Vital Signs**. (*Note:* These findings change over time to reflect the temporal changes you would find in a patient similar to Piya Jordan.)

When you have gathered all the data you need, click on **Patient Care** and then select **Medication Administration**. Any medications you prepared in the previous steps should be listed on the left side of your screen. Let's continue the administration process with the digoxin ordered for Piya Jordan. Click to highlight **Digoxin** in the list of medications. Next, click on the down arrow to the right of **Select** and choose **Administer** from the drop-down menu. This will activate the Administration Wizard. Complete the Wizard sequence as follows:

- Route: **IV**
- Method: **Direct Injection**
- Site: **Peripheral IV**
- Click **Administer to Patient** arrow.
- Would you like to document this administration in the MAR? **Yes**
- Click **Finish** arrow.

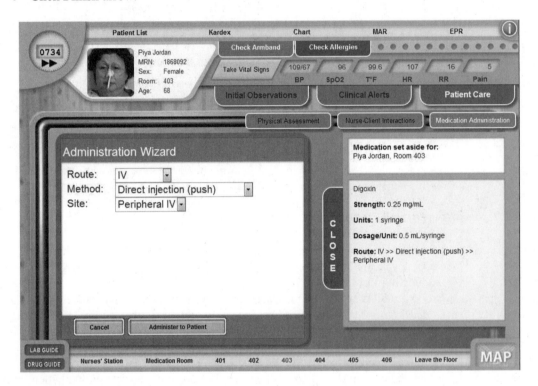

Your selections are recorded by a tracking system and evaluated on a Medication Scorecard stored under Preceptor's Evaluations. This scorecard can be viewed, printed, and given to your instructor. To access the Preceptor's Evaluations, click on **Leave the Floor**. When the Floor Menu appears, select **Preceptor's Evaluation**. Then click on **Medication Scorecard** inside the box with Piya Jordan's name (see example on the following page).

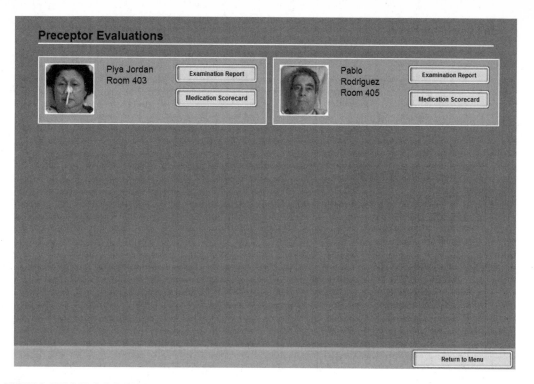

▓ MEDICATION SCORECARD

- First, review Table A. Was digoxin given correctly? Did you give the other medications as ordered?
- Table B shows you which (if any) medications you gave incorrectly.
- Table C addresses the resources used for Piya Jordan. Did you access the patient's chart, MAR, EPR, or Kardex as needed to make safe medication administration decisions?
- Did you check the patient's armband to verify her identity? Did you check whether your patient had any known allergies to medications? Were vital signs taken?

When you have finished reviewing the scorecard, click **Return to Evaluations** and then **Return to Menu**.

■ VITAL SIGNS

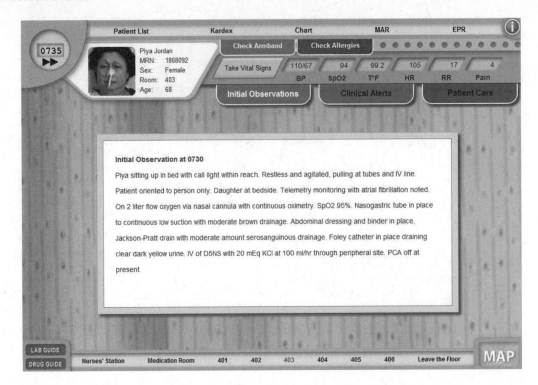

Vital signs, often considered the traditional "signs of life," include body temperature, heart rate, respiratory rate, blood pressure, oxygen saturation of the blood, and pain level.

Inside Piya Jordan's room, click **Take Vital Signs**. (*Note:* If you are following this detailed tour step by step, you will need to **Restart the Program** from the Floor Menu, sign in again for Period of Care 1, and navigate to Room 403.) Collect vital signs for this patient and record them below. Note the time at which you collected each of these data. (*Remember:* You can take vital signs at any time. The data change over time to reflect the temporal changes you would find in a patient similar to Piya Jordan.)

Vital Signs	Findings/Time
Blood pressure	
O₂ saturation	
Temperature	
Heart rate	
Respiratory rate	
Pain rating	

After you are done, click on the **EPR** icon located in the tool bar at the top of the screen. Your username and password are automatically provided. Click on **Login** to enter the EPR. To access Piya Jordan's records, click on the down arrow next to Patient and choose her room number, **403**. Select **Vital Signs** as the category. Next, in the empty time column on the far right, record the vital signs data you just collected in Piya Jordan's room. If you need help with this process, refer to the Electronic Patient Record (EPR) section of **A Quick Tour**. Now compare these findings with the data you collected earlier for this patient's vital signs. Use these earlier findings to establish a baseline for each of the vital signs.

    a. Are any of the data you collected significantly different from the baseline for a particular vital sign?

       Circle One: Yes   No

    b. If "Yes," which data are different?

■ PHYSICAL ASSESSMENT

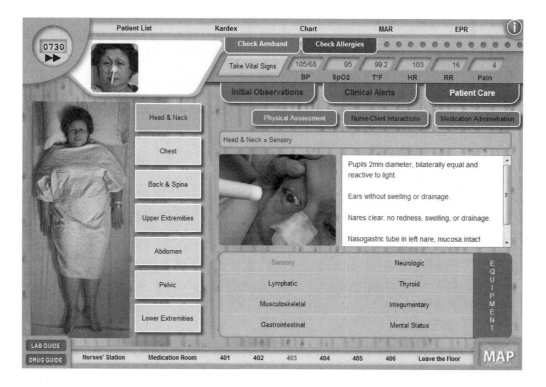

After you have finished examining the EPR for vital signs, click **Exit EPR** to return to Room 403. Click **Patient Care** and then **Physical Assessment**. Think about the information you received in the report at the beginning of this shift, as well as what you may have learned about this patient from the chart. Based on this, what area(s) of examination should you pay most attention to at this time? Is there any equipment you should be monitoring? Conduct a physical assessment of the body areas and systems that you consider priorities for Piya Jordan. For example, select **Head & Neck**; then click on and assess **Sensory** and **Lymphatic**. Complete any other assessment(s) you think are necessary at this time. In the following table, record the data you collected during this examination.

Area of Examination	Findings
Head & Neck Sensory	
Head & Neck Lymphatic	

After you have finished collecting these data, return to the EPR. Compare the data that were already in the record with those you just collected.

a. Are any of the data you collected significantly different from the baselines for this patient?

Circle One: Yes   No

b. If "Yes," which data are different?

■ **NURSE-CLIENT INTERACTIONS**

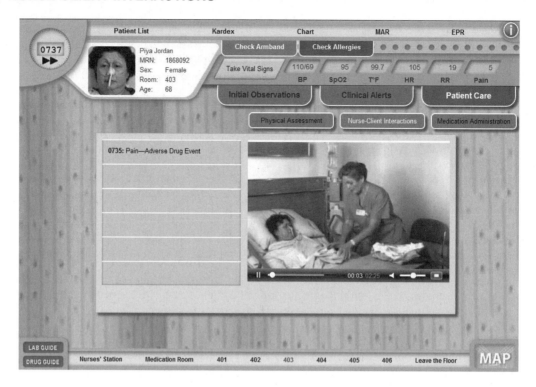

Click on **Patient Care** from inside Piya Jordan's room (403). Now click on **Nurse-Client Interactions** to access a short video titled **Pain—Adverse Drug Event**, which is available for viewing at or after 0735 (based on the virtual clock in the upper left corner of your screen; see *Note* below). To begin the video, click on the white arrow next to its title. You will observe a nurse communicating with Piya Jordan and her daughter. There are many variations of nursing practice, some exemplifying "best" practice and some not. Note whether the nurse in this interaction displays professional behavior and compassionate care. Are her words congruent with what is going on with the patient? Does this interaction "feel right" to you? If not, how would you handle this situation differently? Explain.

Note: If the video you wish to view is not listed, this means you have not yet reached the correct virtual time to view that video. Check the virtual clock; you may return to access the video once its designated time has occurred—as long as you do so within the same period of care. Or you can click on the fast-forward icon within the virtual clock to advance the time by 2-minute intervals. You will then need to click again on **Patient Care** and **Nurse-Client Interactions** to refresh the screen.

At least one Nurse-Client Interactions video is available during each period of care. Viewing these videos can help you learn more about what is occurring with a patient at a certain time and also prompt you to discern between nurse communications that are ideal and those that need improvement. Compassionate care and the ability to communicate clearly are essential components of delivering quality nursing care, and it is during your clinical time that you will begin to refine these skills.

■ COLLECTING AND EVALUATING DATA

Each of the activities you perform in the Patient Care environment generates a significant amount of assessment data. Remember that after you collect data, you can record your findings in the EPR. You can also review the EPR, patient's chart, videos, and MAR at any time. You will get plenty of practice collecting and then evaluating data in context of the patient's course.

Now, here's an important question for you:

> Did the previous sequence of exercises provide the most efficient way to assess Piya Jordan?

For example, you went to the patient's room to get vital signs, then back to the EPR to enter data and compare your findings with extant data. Next, you went back to the patient's room to do a physical examination, then again back to the EPR to enter and review data. If this back-and-forth process of data collection and recording seemed inefficient, remember the following:

- Plan all of your nursing activities to maximize efficiency, while at the same time optimizing the quality of patient care. (Think about what data you might need before performing certain tasks. For example, do you need to check a heart rate before administering a cardiac medication or check an IV site before starting an infusion?)

- You collect a tremendous amount of data when you work with a patient. Very few people can accurately remember all these data for more than a few minutes. Develop efficient assessment skills, and record data as soon as possible after collecting them.

- Assessment data are only the starting point for the nursing process.

Make a clear distinction between these first exercises and how you actually provide nursing care. These initial exercises were designed to involve you actively in the use of different software components. This workbook focuses on sensible practices for implementing the nursing process in ways that ensure the highest-quality care of patients.

Most important, remember that a human being changes through time, and that these changes include both the physical and psychosocial facets of a person as a living organism. Think about this for a moment. Some patients may change physically in a very short time (a patient with emerging myocardial infarction) or more slowly (a patient with a chronic illness). Patients' overall physical and psychosocial conditions may improve or deteriorate. They may have effective coping skills and familial support, or they may feel alone and full of despair. In fact, each individual is a complex mix of physical and psychosocial elements, and at least some of these elements usually change through time.

Thus it is crucial that you *DO NOT* think of the nursing process as a simple one-time, five-step procedure consisting of assessment, nursing diagnosis, planning, implementation, and evaluation. Rather, the nursing process should be utilized as a creative and systematic approach to delivering nursing care. Furthermore, because all living organisms are constantly changing, we must apply the nursing process over and over. Each time we follow the nursing process for an individual patient, we refine our understanding of that patient's physical and psychosocial conditions based on collection and analysis of many different types of data. *Virtual Clinical Excursions—General Hospital* will help you develop both the creativity and the systematic approach needed to become a nurse who is equipped to deliver the highest-quality care to all patients.

REDUCING MEDICATION ERRORS

Earlier in the detailed tour, you learned the basic steps of medication preparation and administration. The following simulations will allow you to practice those skills further—with an increased emphasis on reducing medication errors by using the Medication Scorecard to evaluate your work.

Sign in to work at Pacific View Regional Hospital for Period of Care 1. (*Note:* If you are already working with another patient or during another period of care, click on **Leave the Floor** and then **Restart the Program**; then sign in.)

From the Patient List, select Clarence Hughes. Then click on **Go to Nurses' Station**. Complete the following steps to prepare and administer medications to Clarence Hughes.

- Click on **Medication Room** on the tool bar at the bottom of your screen.
- Click on **MAR** and then on tab **404** to determine medications that have been ordered for Clarence Hughes. (*Note:* You may click on **Review MAR** at any time to verify the correct medication order. Always remember to check the patient name on the MAR to make sure you have the correct patient's record. You must click on the correct room number tab within the MAR.) Click on **Return to Medication Room** after reviewing the correct MAR.
- Click on **Unit Dosage** (or on the Unit Dosage cabinet); from the close-up view, click on drawer **404**.
- Select the medications you would like to administer. After each selection, click **Put Medication on Tray**. When you are finished selecting medications, click **Close Drawer** and then **View Medication Room**.
- Click on **Automated System** (or on the Automated System unit itself). Click **Login**.
- On the next screen, specify the correct patient and drawer location.
- Select the medication you would like to administer and click on **Put Medication on Tray**. Repeat this process if you wish to administer other medications from the Automated System.
- When you are finished, click **Close Drawer** and **View Medication Room**.
- From the Medication Room, click on **Preparation** (or on the preparation tray).
- From the list of medications on your tray, highlight the correct medication to administer and click **Prepare**.
- This activates the Preparation Wizard. Supply any requested information; then click **Next**.
- Now select the correct patient to receive this medication and click **Finish**.
- Repeat the previous three steps until all medications that you want to administer are prepared.
- You can click on **Review Your Medications** and then on **Return to Medication Room** when ready. Once you are back in the Medication Room, go directly to Clarence Hughes' room by clicking on **404** at bottom of screen.
- Inside the patient's room, administer the medication, utilizing the six rights of medication administration. After you have collected the appropriate assessment data and are ready for administration, click **Patient Care** and then **Medication Administration**. Verify that the correct patient and medication(s) appear in the left-hand window. Highlight the first medication you wish to administer; then click the down arrow next to Select. From the drop-down menu, select **Administer** and complete the Administration Wizard by providing any information requested. When the Wizard stops asking for information, click **Administer to Patient**. Specify **Yes** when asked whether this administration should be recorded in the MAR. Finally, click **Finish**.

■ **SELF-EVALUATION**

Now let's see how you did during your medication administration!

- Click on **Leave the Floor** at the bottom of your screen. From the Floor Menu, select **Look at Your Preceptor's Evaluation**. Then click **Medication Scorecard**.

The following exercises will help you identify medication errors, investigate possible reasons for these errors, and reduce or prevent medication errors in the future.

1. Start by examining Table A. These are the medications you should have given to Clarence Hughes during this period of care. If each of the medications in Table A has a ✓ by it, then you made no errors. Congratulations!

If any medication has an X by it, then you made one or more medication errors.

Compare Tables A and B to determine which of the following types of errors you made: Wrong Dose, Wrong Route/Method/Site, or Wrong Time. Follow these steps:
   a. Find medications in Table A that were given incorrectly.
   b. Now see if those same medications are in Table B, which shows what you actually administered to Clarence Hughes.
   c. Comparing Tables A and B, match the Strength, Dose, Route/Method/Site, and Time for each medication you administered incorrectly.
   d. Then, using the form below, list the medications given incorrectly and mark the errors you made for each medication.

Medication	Strength	Dosage	Route	Method	Site	Time
	❑	❑	❑	❑	❑	❑
	❑	❑	❑	❑	❑	❑
	❑	❑	❑	❑	❑	❑
	❑	❑	❑	❑	❑	❑

2. To help you reduce future medication errors, consider the following list of possible reasons for errors.

   - Did not check drug against MAR for correct medication, correct dose, correct patient, correct route, correct time, correct documentation.
   - Did not check drug dose against MAR three times.
   - Did not open the unit dose package in the patient's room.
   - Did not correctly identify the patient using two identifiers.
   - Did not administer the drug on time.
   - Did not verify patient allergies.
   - Did not check the patient's current condition or vital sign parameters.
   - Did not consider why the patient would be receiving this drug.
   - Did not question why the drug was in the patient's drawer.
   - Did not check the physician's order and/or check with the pharmacist when there was a question about the drug or dose.
   - Did not verify that no adverse effects had occurred from a previous dose.

Based on the list of possibilities you just reviewed, determine how you made each error and record the reason in the form below:

Medication	Reason for Error

3. Look again at Table B. Are there medications listed that are not in Table A? If so, you gave a medication to Clarence Hughes that he should not have received. Complete the following exercises to help you understand how such an error might have been made.

   a. Perhaps you gave a medication that was on Clarence Hughes' MAR for this period of care, without recognizing that a change had occurred in the patient's condition, which should have caused you to reconsider. Review patient records as necessary and complete the following form:

Medication	Possible Reasons Not to Give This Medication

   b. Another possibility is that you gave Clarence Hughes a medication that should have been given at a different time. Check his MAR and complete the form below to determine whether you made a Wrong Time error:

Medication	Given to Clarence Hughes at What Time	Should Have Been Given at What Time

c. Maybe you gave another patient's medication to Clarence Hughes. In this case, you made a Wrong Patient error. Check the MARs of other patients and use the form below to determine whether you made this type of error:

Medication	Given to Clarence Hughes	Should Have Been Given to

4. The Medication Scorecard provides some other interesting sources of information. For example, if there is a medication selected for Clarence Hughes but it was not given to him, there will be an X by that medication in Table A, but it will not appear in Table B. In that case, you might have given this medication to some other patient, which is another type of Wrong Patient error. To investigate further, look at Table D, which lists the medications you gave to other patients. See whether you can find any medications ordered for Clarence Hughes that were given to another patient by mistake. However, before you make any decisions, be sure to cross-check the MAR for other patients because the same medication may have been ordered for multiple patients. Use the following form to record your findings:

Medication	Should Have Been Given to Clarence Hughes	Given by Mistake to

5. Now take some time to review the medication exercises you just completed. Use the form below to create an overall analysis of what you have learned. Once again, record each of the medication errors you made, including the type of each error. Then, for each error you made, indicate specifically what you would do differently to prevent this type of error from occurring again.

Medication	Type of Error	Error Prevention Tactic

Submit this form to your instructor if required as a graded assignment, or simply use these exercises to improve your understanding of medication errors and how to reduce them.

Name: _____   Date: _____

Priority Setting and Goal Development

Reading Assignment: Concepts of Health, Illness, Stress, and Health Promotion (Chapter 2)
The Nursing Process and Critical Thinking (Chapter 4)
Assessment, Nursing Diagnosis, and Planning (Chapter 5)
Concepts of Basic Nutrition and Cultural Considerations (Chapter 26)

Patient: Patricia Newman, Medical-Surgical Floor, Room 406

Objectives:

1. Prioritize nursing diagnoses in order of importance for a patient's well-being.
2. Prioritize tasks appropriately.
3. Develop individualized patient outcomes.

Exercise 1

Writing Activity: Patient Needs

5 minutes

1. Identify the eight needs categories that must be considered when performing an assessment (data collection) on a patient.

Exercise 2

Virtual Hospital Activity—Problems and Nursing Diagnoses

15 minutes

- Sign in to work at Pacific View Regional Hospital on the Medical-Surgical Floor for Period of Care 3. (*Note:* If you are already in the virtual hospital from a previous exercise, click on **Leave the Floor** and then on **Restart the Program** to get to the sign-in window.)
- From the Patient List, select Patricia Newman (Room 406).
- Click on **Get Report** and read the report. (*Note:* When you read this report, you will see terms such as "decreased FEV" and some "ABG" results. In case these terms are unfamiliar to you, these diagnostic results indicate the patient is experiencing respiratory distress.)
- Click on **Go to Nurses' Station**.
- Click on **EPR** and then on **Login**.
- Specify **406** from the Patient drop-down menu and **Nutrition** from the Category drop-down menu.

  1. Patricia Newman ate _____% of her breakfast and _____% of her lunch.

- Click on **Exit EPR**.
- Next, click on **Chart** and then on **406**.
- Click on **Consultations** and read the Dietary Consult.

  2. What are the dietary recommendations made by the dietitian?

  3. Below, match each nursing diagnosis with the related problem area.

Problem Area	Nursing Diagnosis
_____ Discharge	a. Decreased gas exchange
_____ Fluid/volume electrolyte imbalance	b. Need for health teaching
_____ Infection	c. Inadequate nutrition
_____ Nutrition	d. Hyperthermia
_____ Respiratory	e. Potential infection
_____ Thermoregulation	f. Fluid overload

4. Below, match each piece of data with the patient problem it supports.

Patient Problem	Data
_____ Decreased gas exchange	a. Is eating 30% to 40% of meals
_____ Inadequate nutrition	b. Tires easily
_____ Decreased adherence	c. Temperature 102.5 degrees F
_____ Need for health teaching	d. Crackles in lower lobes of lungs
_____ Hyperthermia	e. Is removing nasal oxygen cannula

5. What elements and considerations would be used in prioritizing nursing diagnoses for Patricia Newman?

6. The following patient problems apply to Patricia Newman. Match the columns to put them in priority order (with 1 being the highest priority).

Patient Problem	Order of Priority
_____ Decreased gas exchange	a. 1
_____ Need for health teaching	b. 2
_____ Inadequate nutrition	c. 3

Exercise 3

Virtual Hospital Activity—Priorities Based on Maslow's Hierarchy

30 minutes

- Sign in to work at Pacific View Regional Hospital on the Medical-Surgical Floor for Period of Care 3. (*Note:* If you are already in the virtual hospital from a previous exercise, click on **Leave the Floor** and then on **Restart the Program** to get to the sign-in window.)
- From the Patient List, select Patricia Newman (Room 406).
- Click on **Go to Nurses' Station** and then on **406** at the bottom of the screen.
- Read the Initial Observations.
- Click on **Chart** and then on **406**.
- Click on and review the **Nursing Admission**.

1. a. What is Patricia Newman's height? _____

   b. What is her weight? _____

   c. What is her age? _____

2. Do you think that Patricia Newman's weight is appropriate for her height and age?

3. If the nurse will assist with data collection by performing a focused assessment, what should be the focus of the assessment?

4. Besides the fact that Patricia Newman is eating only small portions of her meals, what other data have you gathered that support the nursing diagnosis of inadequate nutrition? Select all that apply.

_____   5 ft 5 in tall; weight 120 lb

_____   Fatigues easily

_____   Has frequent infections

_____   Needs supplemental oxygen

5. Considering the dietitian's recommendations, Patricia Newman's respiratory status, and her diagnosis of pneumonia, select the action that would be the first priority for her. (*Hint:* Read about pneumonia in your medical-surgical textbook if you need help.)

_____   Explain the importance of keeping the oxygen cannula in place.

_____   Return the oxygen cannula to her nose.

_____   Encourage her to drink 8 oz of water.

_____   Assess what liquids she finds appealing.

_____   Discuss why she should eat more of her meals.

6. Now select the next priority action for Patricia Newman.

_____   Explain the importance of keeping the oxygen cannula in place.

_____   Return the oxygen cannula to her nose.

_____   Encourage her to drink 8 oz of water.

_____   Assess what liquids she finds appealing.

_____   Discuss why she should eat more of her meals.

7. Which of the following would be considered first-level needs for Patricia Newman, according to Maslow's hierarchy? Select all that apply.

_____ Hygiene

_____ Rest and comfort

_____ Psychologic comfort

_____ Affection

_____ Activity

_____ Elimination

_____ Safety

_____ Sexual procreation

_____ Intimacy

_____ Achievement

_____ Learning

Critical Thinking and Problem Solving

Reading Assignment: The Nursing Process and Critical Thinking (Chapter 4)
Assessment, Nursing Diagnosis, and Planning (Chapter 5)
Assisting with Respiration and Oxygen Delivery (Chapter 28)

Patient: Patricia Newman, Medical-Surgical Floor, Room 406

Objectives:

1. Use critical thinking to gather and analyze data presented in the case study.
2. Use the problem-solving process to decide which assessment data are needed to provide appropriate nursing care for a patient.
3. Use critical thinking in order to organize tasks and set priorities.

Exercise 1

Virtual Hospital Activity—Gathering Data

15 minutes

- Sign in to work at Pacific View Regional Hospital on the Medical-Surgical Floor for Period of Care 1. (*Note:* If you are already in the virtual hospital from a previous exercise, click on **Leave the Floor** and then on **Restart the Program** to get to the sign-in window.)
- From the Patient List, select Patricia Newman (Room 406).
- Click on **Get Report** and read the report.
- Click on **Go to Nurses' Station**.
- Click on **Chart** and then on **406**. Review the **Physician's Notes** and **Nursing Admission**.

1. Using the change-of-shift report, fill in the following information for Patricia Newman.

   Respiratory status: _____

   Vital signs:

   • Blood pressure _____

   • Heart rate _____

   • Respiratory rate _____

   • Temperature _____

   • Oxygen saturation _____

   IV: _____

   Priority problem: _____

   Diagnostic tests: _____

2. Which of the following sections of Patricia Newman's patient records will you need to consult at this time to gather necessary data to safely care for her? Select all that apply.

   _____ Admissions Records

   _____ Operative Reports

   _____ Nursing History

   _____ Medication Records

   _____ History and Physical

   _____ Social Services

   _____ Physician's Notes

   _____ Nurse's Notes

   _____ Diagnostic Reports

   _____ Kardex

   _____ Physician's Orders

• Click on **Return to Nurses' Station**.
• Click on **Kardex** at the top of the screen. Click on **406** and read Patricia Newman's records. (*Remember:* The Kardex provides access to the records of all patients on the floor—not just the patient for whom you are currently caring. Be sure you are looking at the Kardex for the correct room number.)

3. Does Patricia Newman have any allergies that are pertinent to your care for her?

4. What categories of problems are marked "initiated" on Patricia Newman's Kardex?

5. What are Patricia Newman's diagnoses, as listed on the Kardex?

6. Which area is the priority problem for Patricia Newman at this time?

_____ Movement and activity

_____ Circulation

_____ Airway and breathing

_____ Safety

_____ Security

_____ Elimination

Exercise 2

Virtual Hospital Activity—Priority Assessments and Pulse Oximetry

30 minutes

- Sign in to work at Pacific View Regional Hospital on the Medical-Surgical Floor for Period of Care 1. (*Note:* If you are already in the virtual hospital from a previous exercise, click on **Leave the Floor** and then on **Restart the Program** to get to the sign-in window.)
- From the Patient List, select Patricia Newman (Room 406).
- Click on **Go to Nurses' Station**.
- Click on **Chart** and then on **406**.
- Click on **Physician's Orders**.

1. What is the physician's order for frequency of measuring the patient's vital signs and oxygen saturation?

2. Considering Patricia Newman's respiratory status and problems, determine assessments that should be performed during your first visit to the patient. Below, select all the areas you would prioritize on your first visit to Patricia Newman.

_____ Vital signs

_____ Verbal complaints

_____ Heart

_____ Lungs

_____ IV

_____ Eyes

_____ Pain level

_____ Skin

_____ Extremities

_____ Abdomen

_____ Neurologic status

- Click on **Return to Nurses' Station**.
- Now click on **406** at the bottom of your screen to go to Patricia Newman's room.
- Read the Initial Observations and then click on and read the **Clinical Alerts**.

3. What concerns are highlighted in the Initial Observations and the Clinical Alerts notes?

- Click on **Check Armband** and then on **Take Vital Signs**.

4. Record Patricia Newman's vital sign measurements below. (*Note:* You will need to enter them in the EPR later.)

Blood pressure _____

Temperature _____

Oxygen saturation _____

Heart rate _____

Respiratory rate _____

Pain level _____

Read about pulse oximetry in your textbook.

5. How does the pulse oximeter measure oxygen saturation?

6. Is there a problem with using a fingertip probe for pulse oximetry if the patient is wearing nail polish or artificial nails?

7. What other elements may impede assessment with the pulse oximeter?

8. It is not possible to use Patricia Newman's finger for the pulse oximeter probe, where else could you place the probe?

9. Normal SpO_2 is _____ to _____.

• Click on **Patient Care** and then on **Chest**.
• Click on **Respiratory** and note the respiratory assessment data.
• Click on **Musculoskeletal** and note the data that are pertinent regarding respiration.

10. Record the respiratory assessment findings below.

• Click on **Chart** and then on **406**.
• Click on **Emergency Department** and review.
• Click on **Nurse's Notes** and read all previous notes.

11. Using the information found in the chart and the data collected during patient assessment, indicate which symptoms of hypoxia Patricia Newman has had. Select all that apply.

_____ Nausea

_____ Using accessory muscles to breathe

_____ Stating "I'm really short of breath"

_____ Cyanosis

_____ Tachypnea

_____ Tachycardia

_____ Hypothermia

- Click on **Return to Room 406**.
- Click on **EPR** and then on **Login**.
- Choose **406** from the Patient drop-down menu and **Vital Signs** from the Category drop-down menu.
- In the correct column, enter the pain rating and vital signs you recorded in question 4 of this exercise.
- Now choose **Respiratory** from the Category drop-down menu. Enter the data you obtained when that system was assessed in question 10 of this exercise.
- Click on the various fields where data are entered to highlight and view the codes used for that part of the system. (*Hint:* The code meanings are listed to the right of the data columns.)

12. What differences did you find between what you just charted and what was charted for these systems on Wednesday at 0300?

Exercise 3

Virtual Hospital Activity—Problem Solving and Prioritizing

15 minutes

- Sign in to work at Pacific View Regional Hospital on the Medical-Surgical Floor for Period of Care 1. (*Note:* If you are already in the virtual hospital from a previous exercise, click on **Leave the Floor** and then on **Restart the Program** to get to the sign-in window.)
- From the Patient List, select Patricia Newman (Room 406).
- Click on **Go to Nurses' Station**.

1. Which area is the priority problem for Patricia Newman at this time?
   a. Movement and activity
   b. Circulation
   c. Airway and oxygenation
   d. Safety
   e. Security

2. What are priority assessments to make for Patricia Newman's safety needs while she is using oxygen?

3. Patricia Newman has obstructive lung disease and should have her oxygen concentration limited to

   only _____ to _____ L/min.

4. You will be expected to do discharge teaching for Patricia Newman during her hospital stay. Review
   the actions listed below and number them in order of priority (with 1 being the highest priority).

Action	**Order of Priority**
_____ Provide smoking cessation literature to the patient.	a. 1
_____ Find out how she feels about the repeated hospitalizations.	b. 2
	c. 3
_____ Ask whether she has ever tried to quit smoking.	
	d. 4
_____ Explain how smoking predisposes her to lung infection.	e. 5
_____ Provide a list of community resources for help with quitting smoking.	

5. If Patricia Newman's respiratory status deteriorates, which signs of early hypoxia and respiratory
   insufficiency would the nurse possibly detect?

Exercise 4

Virtual Hospital Activity—Interventions to Meet Expected Outcomes

15 minutes

- Sign in to work at Pacific View Regional Hospital on the Medical-Surgical Floor for Period of Care 1. (*Note:* If you are already in the virtual hospital from a previous exercise, click on **Leave the Floor** and then on **Restart the Program** to get to the sign-in window.)
- From the Patient List, select Patricia Newman (Room 406).
- Click on **Go to Nurses' Station**.
- Click on **MAR** and then on tab **406** to view Patricia Newman's MAR. Scroll down to the second page of the MAR.

1. Atenolol has been ordered to manage Patricia Newman's hypertension. What impact will this medication have on her cardiac output and heart rate? (*Hint:* Refer to the Drug Guide.)

2. Indicate whether the following statement is true or false.

   _____ Atenolol will increase the myocardial oxygen demand.

3. When preparing to administer atenolol, which of the following nursing actions is indicated? Select all that apply.

   _____ Measure the patient's temperature.

   _____ Measure the apical pulse.

   _____ Measure the blood pressure.

   _____ Assess respirations.

   _____ Check renal function and liver function laboratory results.

   _____ Auscultate lung fields.

Communication and the Nurse-Patient Relationship

Reading Assignment: Documentation of Nursing Care (Chapter 7)
Communication and the Nurse-Patient Relationship (Chapter 8)

Patients: Harry George, Medical-Surgical Floor, Room 401
Clarence Hughes, Medical-Surgical Floor, Room 404
William Jefferson, Skilled Nursing Unit, Room 501

Objectives:

1. List the factors that influence the way a person communicates.
2. Differentiate effective communication techniques from those that block communication.
3. Identify effective techniques to gather information from patients.
4. Document patient care appropriately.

Exercise 1

Virtual Hospital Activity—Communication Skills

30 minutes

- Sign in to work at Pacific View Regional Hospital on the Medical-Surgical Floor for Period of Care 1. (*Note:* If you are already in the virtual hospital from a previous exercise, click on **Leave the Floor** and then on **Restart the Program** to get to the sign-in window.)
- From the Patient List, select Harry George (Room 401).
- Click on **Get Report**.
- Read the report and note any data indicating a possible problem.
- Click on **Go to Nurses' Station** and then on **401** to visit the patient's room.
- Click on **Patient Care** and then on **Nurse-Client Interactions**.
- Select and view the video titled **0735: Symptom Management**. (*Note:* Check the virtual clock to see whether enough time has elapsed. You can use the fast-forward feature to advance the time by 2-minute intervals if the video is not yet available. Then click again on **Patient Care** and **Nurse-Client Interactions** to refresh the screen.)

1. Review Harry George's nonverbal behavior during the exchange with the sitter. Describe what you observe for each of the elements listed below.

Personal appearance

Facial expression

Eye contact

2. Review the sitter's response to Harry George's complaints. Which of the following communication techniques does he attempt to employ?
   a. Restating
   b. Clarifying
   c. Touch
   d. Summarizing

3. Indicate whether the following statement is true or false.

   _____ During the interaction between Harry George and the sitter, the patient's nonverbal behavior was consistent with his spoken comments.

4. Harry George is anxious. How can anxiety affect communication?

5. The term _____ is used to describe an inconsistency between verbal and nonverbal behaviors.

6. During the interaction, the nurse approaches Harry George and inquires about his level of pain and the effectiveness of the analgesics given. Describe the nurse's entry into the patient's personal space. Was it appropriate?

7. When communicating with patients, the nurse should be aware of the cultural influences on social distance. Which groups traditionally maintain more distance from others when communicating? Select all that apply.

_____ American Indians

_____ Asians

_____ Hispanics

_____ Middle Eastern

_____ Northern Europeans

_____ Southern European

8. As the nurse begins the conversation with Harry George, she asks him about the effectiveness of his

pain medication. The nurse phrases this as a(n) _____-ended question.

9. After Harry George expressed his belief that alcohol would make him feel better, the nurse responded by providing him with education related to the dangers of his behavior. Was this the appropriate response by the nurse? What factors should the nurse pay close attention to when providing such information?

10. Review the nurse's interaction with Harry George. Do you have any concerns about the manner in which the nurse interacted with him?

11. Compare and contrast the report from the Initial Observations at 0730 and Harry George's demeanor during the 0735 Nurse-Client Interaction video.

12. To demonstrate empathy for Harry George, which of the following would be appropriate? Select all that apply.

_____ Reflection of the patient's expressed thoughts

_____ Focus on the patient's feelings

_____ Very close physical proximity to the patient

_____ A warm tone of voice

_____ Suggestions on how to best solve the patient's problems

_____ A nonjudgmental attitude

- Click on **Patient Care** and then on **Nurse-Client Interactions**.
- Select and view the video titled **0755: Disease Management**. (*Note:* Check the virtual clock to see whether enough time has elapsed. You can use the fast-forward feature to advance the time by 2-minute intervals if the video is not yet available. Then click again on **Patient Care** and **Nurse-Client Interactions** to refresh the screen.)

13. In response to Harry George's complaints of pain, which of the following communication techniques is being employed by the sitter?
    a. Empathy
    b. Restatement
    c. Distraction
    d. Touch

- Click on **Patient Care** and then on **Nurse-Client Interactions**.
- Select and view the video titled **0810: The Patient in Pain**. (*Note:* Check the virtual clock to see whether enough time has elapsed. You can use the fast-forward feature to advance the time by 2-minute intervals if the video is not yet available. Then click again on **Patient Care** and **Nurse-Client Interactions** to refresh the screen.)

14. Compare the sitter's demeanor in this interaction with that in the earlier (0735) video. Which do you think is more appropriate?

Exercise 2

Virtual Hospital Activity—Communication Techniques

30 minutes

- Sign in to work at Pacific View Regional Hospital on the Skilled Nursing Floor for Period of Care 1. (*Note:* If you are already in the virtual hospital from a previous exercise, click on **Leave the Floor** and then on **Restart the Program** to get to the sign-in window.)
- From the Patient List, select William Jefferson (Room 501).
- Click on **Get Report** and read the report.
- Click on **Go to Nurses' Station**.
- Click on **Chart** and then on **501**.
- Click on and review the **History and Physical**.
- Click on **Return to Nurses' Station** and then on **501** to go to the patient's room.
- Read the Initial Observations.

1. What psychosocial issues could affect the nurse's communication with William Jefferson? How might these behaviors affect the interaction?

2. What physiologic and environmental issues being experienced by William Jefferson may affect the nurse-patient interaction?

3. Which of the following interventions will assist the nurse in establishing a positive rapport when communicating with William Jefferson? Select all that apply.

   _____ Assist the patient to the dining room to promote feelings of socialization.

   _____ Face him during interactions.

   _____ Avoid analgesic administration to reduce drowsiness during interactions.

   _____ Provide adequate lighting during interactions.

   _____ Use touch as culturally appropriate.

4. When the nurse is caring for William Jefferson, which of the following variables will have the most influence on communication?
   a. Patient's age and race
   b. Patient's culture and social position
   c. Scheduled agenda for the day
   d. Race of the care provider
   e. Disorientation and confusion

- Click on **Patient Care** and then on **Nurse-Client Interactions**.
- Select and view the video titled **0730: Intervention—Patient Safety**. (*Note:* Check the virtual clock to see whether enough time has elapsed. You can use the fast-forward feature to advance the time by 2-minute intervals if the video is not yet available. Then click again on **Patient Care** and **Nurse-Client Interactions** to refresh the screen.)

5. Review and critique the nurse's interaction with William Jefferson. What behaviors indicate that the nurse is attempting to establish a rapport with him?

6. Which of the following is the primary concern for the nurse during the interaction?

   _____ The safety of the patient

   _____ The patient's disorientation

   _____ Locating the patient's family members

   _____ The patient's ability to tolerate ambulation

- Click on **Patient Care** and then on **Nurse-Client Interactions**.
- Select and view the video titled **0740: The Confused Patient**. (*Note:* Check the virtual clock to see whether enough time has elapsed. You can use the fast-forward feature to advance the time by 2-minute intervals if the video is not yet available. Then click again on **Patient Care** and **Nurse-Client Interactions** to refresh the screen.)

7. During the interaction, what communication techniques are used by the nurse?

8. The nurse's initial attempts to touch William Jefferson are rebuffed. Are repeated attempts appropriate?

9. Review William Jefferson's appearance and behaviors during the exchange. List your findings for each area below.

Personal appearance

Facial expression

Eye contact

- Click on **Patient Care** and then on **Nurse-Client Interactions**.
- Select and view the video titled **0745: Intervention—Redirection**. (*Note:* Check the virtual clock to see whether enough time has elapsed. You can use the fast-forward feature to advance the time by 2-minute intervals if the video is not yet available. Then click again on **Patient Care** and **Nurse-Client Interactions** to refresh the screen.)

10. What is the primary underlying purpose of the communication technique being demonstrated by the nurse during the interaction?
    a. Distraction
    b. Assessment of patient's cognition
    c. Assessment of patient's personal interests
    d. Evaluation of patient's needs

11. How does William Jefferson's demeanor and interaction with the nurse in this exchange differ from the previous interaction?

Exercise 3

Virtual Hospital Activity—Therapeutic Communication and Empathy

30 minutes

- Sign in to work at Pacific View Regional Hospital on the Medical-Surgical Floor for Period of Care 1. (*Note:* If you are already in the virtual hospital from a previous exercise, click on **Leave the Floor** and then on **Restart the Program** to get to the sign-in window.)
- From the Patient List, select Clarence Hughes (Room 404).
- Click on **Get Report**.
- Read the report and note any data indicating a possible problem.
- Click on **Go to Nurses' Station** and then on **404** to visit the patient's room.
- Click on **Patient Care** and then on **Nurse-Client Interactions**.

- Select and view the video titled **0730: Assessment/Perception of Care**. (*Note:* Check the virtual clock to see whether enough time has elapsed. You can use the fast-forward feature to advance the time by 2-minute intervals if the video is not yet available. Then click again on **Patient Care** and **Nurse-Client Interactions** to refresh the screen.)

1. What nonverbal actions and/or signs did you observe while watching Clarence Hughes?

2. Do the nonverbal messages agree with what Clarence Hughes is saying to the nurse?

3. Do you think it is appropriate for the nurse to ask to do the assessment before giving Clarence Hughes the pain medication he is requesting? Why or why not?

- Click on **Patient Care** and then on **Nurse-Client Interactions**.
- Select and view the video titled **0735: Empathy**. (*Note:* Check the virtual clock to see whether enough time has elapsed. You can use the fast-forward feature to advance the time by 2-minute intervals if the video is not yet available. Then click again on **Patient Care** and **Nurse-Client Interactions** to refresh the screen.)

4. Was the nurse's first question to Clarence Hughes therapeutic or nontherapeutic? What type of technique did the nurse use by asking this question?

Read about continuous passive motion (CPM) in your textbook.

5. Is the nurse showing empathy for Clarence Hughes' pain of 8/10 when she says she will put the CPM back on after giving him his pain medication?

6. Which of the following are elements of empathy? Select all that apply.

_____ Reflection of the person's expressed thought

_____ Focus on the person's feelings

_____ Very close physical proximity

_____ Warm tone of voice

_____ Suggestions on how to solve the problem

_____ A nonjudgmental attitude

- Still in Clarence Hughes' room, click on **Initial Observations** and read the note.
- Now click on **Clinical Alerts** and read the note.
- Click on **Take Vital Signs**.

7. Record Clarence Hughes' vital signs below.

Blood pressure _____

Temperature _____

Oxygen saturation _____

Heart rate _____

Respiratory rate _____

Pain level _____

- Click on **Patient Care** and then on **Physical Assessment**.
- Click on **Lower Extremities** and conduct a focused assessment on Clarence Hughes by clicking on each of the subcategories (green buttons). (*Note:* Jot down pertinent findings so that you will be able to document the assessment later.)

8. Using your assessment data and the information from the video interactions, write a SOAP note below regarding Clarence Hughes' pain and surgical site (*Note:* Write this note just as you would for the patient's chart.)

S

O

A

P

- Click on **EPR** in the upper right area of the screen. Click on **Login**.
- Select **404** from the Patient drop-down menu and **Vital Signs** from the Category drop-down menu.
- In the correct column, enter the vital signs and pain assessment data you obtained during this exercise. Highlight each pertinent line to view the codes and meanings available to you.
- Click on **Exit EPR** and then on **Chart**. Click on **404** and select **Nurse's Notes**.
- Read the note relevant to the 0730 Nurse-Client Interaction you observed earlier.

9. What type of documentation did the nurse use to write this nurse's note?

_____ POMR

_____ DAR

_____ PIE

_____ Focus charting

_____ Narrative charting

_____ Charting by exception

10. Is the information obtained from Clarence Hughes about his pain subjective or objective data? Explain.

Documentation of Nursing Care

Reading Assignment: Documentation of Nursing Care (Chapter 7)

Patients: Harry George, Medical-Surgical Floor, Room 401
Clarence Hughes, Medical-Surgical Floor, Room 404

Objectives:

1. Document patient care in electronic patient records.
2. Identify data that should be documented in the nurse's notes.
3. Correctly document in the nurse's notes.
4. List data that should be included when documenting a change in condition.

Exercise 1

Virtual Hospital Activity—Exploring Documentation

30 minutes

- Sign in to work at Pacific View Regional Hospital on the Medical-Surgical Floor for Period of Care 2. (*Note:* If you are already in the virtual hospital from a previous exercise, click on **Leave the Floor** and then on **Restart the Program** to get to the sign-in window.)
- From the Patient List, select Clarence Hughes (Room 404).
- Click on **Get Report** and review.
- Click on **Go to Nurses' Station** and then on **404**.
- Inside the patient's room, click on **Take Vital Signs**.

1. Record Clarence Hughes' current vital signs below.

   Blood pressure _____

   Oxygen saturation _____

   Temperature _____

   Heart rate _____

   Respiratory rate _____

   Pain level _____

- Read the Initial Observations.
- Click on **Clinical Alerts** and read the note.
- Click on **Patient Care** and then on **Nurse-Client Interactions**.
- Select and view the video titled **1115: Interventions—Airway**. (*Note:* Check the virtual clock to see whether enough time has elapsed. You can use the fast-forward feature to advance the time by 2-minute intervals if the video is not yet available. Then click again on **Patient Care** and **Nurse-Client Interactions** to refresh the screen.)
- Now click on **Patient Care** and then on **Physical Assessment**.
- Click on **Chest** and then on each subcategory for the chest assessment, noting any abnormal data.
- Click on **EPR** and then on **Login**.
- Select **404** from the Patient drop-down menu and **Vital Signs** from the Category drop-down menu.
- In the correct column, enter the vital sign data you obtained in question 1.
- Now select **Respiratory** from the Category drop-down menu. Enter the data you obtained during that portion of the chest assessment. Highlight each line to see the codes and meanings you may use for that specific item.
- Next, choose **Cardiovascular** and enter that assessment data.
- Finally, select **Psychosocial** and enter the data regarding Clarence Hughes' anxiety.
- Return to the **Vital Signs** category.

2. Which vital sign measurements have changed considerably since they were last taken? Select all that apply.

_____ Blood pressure

_____ Temperature

_____ Heart rate

_____ Oxygen saturation

_____ Respiratory rate

3. What nonverbal communication did you observe in the video interaction that indicated Clarence Hughes is in distress?

4. Below, using a focus charting format, write a nurse's note regarding the change in Clarence Hughes' condition.

D

A

R

- Before leaving the EPR, familiarize yourself with the various available charting sections of this electronic format by choosing each category in turn and reviewing the data lines available for that area.
- Now click on **Exit EPR** and then on **Chart**.
- Select **404** and click on **Nurse's Notes**.
- Compare the nurse's note in the chart with the note you wrote for question 4.

5. Did you omit anything important from the nurse's note you wrote for question 4?

Exercise 2

Virtual Hospital Activity—Documentation Practice

45 minutes

- Sign in to work at Pacific View Regional Hospital on the Medical-Surgical Floor for Period of Care 1. (*Note:* If you are already in the virtual hospital from a previous exercise, click on **Leave the Floor** and then on **Restart the Program** to get to the sign-in window.)
- From the Patient List, select Harry George (Room 401).
- Click on **Get Report** and read the report.
- Click on **Go to Nurses' Station** and then on **401** to go to Harry George's room.
- Read the Initial Observations.
- Click on **Clinical Alerts** to determine whether there is an immediate nursing need.
- Click on **Take Vital Signs**.

1. What are Harry George's current vital signs?

   Blood pressure _____

   Oxygen saturation _____

   Temperature _____

   Heart rate _____

   Respiratory rate _____

   Pain level _____

- Begin a brief assessment on Harry George by clicking on **Patient Care** and then on **Physical Assessment**.
- Next, click on **Head & Neck** from the body system categories (yellow buttons) and then on **Mental Status** from the subcategories (green buttons).

2. What is Harry George's current mental status?

- Click on **Lower Extremities** and then on each of the available subcategories.
- Make note of any pertinent findings for later entry in the EPR or for writing a nurse's note.

3. What do your findings from the assessment of Harry George's lower extremities reveal?

- Click on **EPR** in the right corner of the screen and then click on **Login**.
- Select **401** from the Patient drop-down menu and **Vital Signs** from the Category drop-down menu.
- Locate the Wed 0730 time column. Record your vital signs findings from question 1.
- Now choose **Cardiovascular** from the Category drop-down menu and enter the data you obtained from the vascular assessment of the lower extremities.
- Next, select **Neurologic** and enter the data you obtained regarding Harry George's mental status.

- Choose **Musculoskeletal** and enter the data you obtained when you assessed the lower extremities.
- Select **Integumentary** and enter the appropriate code for the assessment of the lower extremities.
- Finally, select **Wounds and Drains** and enter the codes for the assessment of Harry George's leg wound.

4. Now write a nurse's note for the remaining assessment data that you could not record in the EPR. Use source-oriented or narrative charting.

- Click on **Exit EPR**.
- Click on **Chart** and then on **401**.
- Click on **Physician's Orders**. Find the order for pain medication.

5. The medication order written for Harry George's pain is

_____.

- Click on **Return to Room 401** and then on **MAR**. Select tab **401** and search for the pain medication you found in the physician's order.

6. Harry George received the new pain medication at _____.

- Click on **Return to Room 401**.
- Click on **Chart** and then **401**.
- Click on the **Nurse's Notes** and read the note for the beginning of this shift.

7. What does the nurse's note say about Harry George's pain level and administration of pain medication?

Exercise 3

Virtual Hospital Activity—Other Charting Formats

30 minutes

- Sign in to work at Pacific View Regional Hospital on the Medical-Surgical Floor for Period of Care 1. (*Note:* If you are already in the virtual hospital from a previous exercise, click on **Leave the Floor** and then on **Restart the Program** to get to the sign-in window.)
- From the Patient List, select Harry George (Room 401).
- Click on **Go to Nurses' Station**.

1. Match each piece of data below with its correct data type.

Data	Data Type
_____ "My pain is at 8/10."	a. Subjective
_____ Left lower leg erythematous from toes to mid-calf.	b. Objective
_____ "It hurts to move my foot."	
_____ Serous drainage from wound.	
_____ Temperature 100.2 degrees F.	
_____ "Bring me my bottle and a cigarette."	

2. Match each piece of assessment data listed below with the location in the patient record where it should be documented.

Data Obtained	Where to Document Data
_____ Open lesion 2-3 cm on left ankle	a. Chart only
_____ Right pedal pulse 2+	b. EPR only
_____ Pain at 6/10	c. Chart and EPR
_____ Skin erythematous from toes to mid-calf of left leg	
_____ Impaired ROM in left leg	
_____ Asking for alcohol and cigarettes	
_____ Alert and oriented to person, place, and situation	
_____ Hydromorphone 2 mg IV given at 0715	

3. Unless documented to the contrary, the charting by exception format assumes that:
   a. the body system was assessed.
   b. data obtained are irrelevant.
   c. all standards and protocols were followed.
   d. a full physical assessment has been performed.

4. Which of the following are true of the charting guidelines for correct, legally accurate documentation? Select all that apply.

_____ Use only agency-accepted symbols and abbreviations in documentation.

_____ Visitors should be mentioned by name.

_____ Physician visits should be documented.

_____ Start each sentence with a capital letter and end with a period.

_____ Use complete sentences when documenting in the nurse's notes.

_____ When the patient is the subject of the sentence, leave "patient" out of the sentence.

_____ Do not duplicate the charting of an item on a flow sheet in the nurse's notes.

_____ Chart only what you have performed or observed.

_____ Pencil may be used on a flow sheet.

_____ Entries must not be erased or covered with any type of correction fluid.

• Click on **401** to go to the patient's room.
• Click on **Patient Care** and then on **Nurse-Client Interactions**.
• Select and view the video titled **0810: The Patient in Pain**. (*Note:* Check the virtual clock to see whether enough time has elapsed. You can use the fast-forward feature to advance the time by 2-minute intervals if the video is not yet available. Then click again on **Patient Care** and **Nurse-Client Interactions** to refresh the screen.)

5. Below, write a SOAP note regarding the interaction you just observed between the patient and the sitter.

S

O

A

P

6. PIE charting is another style of charting. Using the PIE format, document the interaction you observed between the patient and the sitter.

P

I

E

Patient Teaching

Reading Assignment: Patient Education and Health Promotion (Chapter 9)

Patients: Piya Jordan, Medical-Surgical Floor, Room 403
Clarence Hughes, Medical-Surgical Floor, Room 404
Patricia Newman, Medical-Surgical Floor, Room 406

Objectives:

1. Identify areas of the need for health teaching for patients.
2. Recognize factors that may affect learning for individual patients.
3. Determine the best methods for teaching specific content.
4. Devise individualized teaching plans.

Exercise 1

Virtual Hospital Activity—Assessing Learning Needs

30 minutes

- Sign in to work at Pacific View Regional Hospital on the Medical-Surgical Floor for Period of Care 3. (*Note:* If you are already in the virtual hospital from a previous exercise, click on **Leave the Floor** and then on **Restart the Program** to get to the sign-in window.)
- From the Patient List, select Patricia Newman (Room 406).
- Click on **Go to Nurses' Station**.
- Click on **Chart** and then on **406**.
- Click on the **Nursing Admission**.

1. What factors mentioned in the chart do you think may interfere with learning for Patricia Newman at this time? Select all that apply.

_____ Pain

_____ Fatigue

_____ Fever

_____ Anxiety

_____ Decreased oxygenation

_____ Nausea

_____ Sedation

_____ Visitor

Review the Modes of Learning and Factors Affecting Learning in your textbook.

2. Based on your review of the Nursing Admission assessment, you determine that Patricia Newman most likely learns best by what type of instructions? This means she is what kind of learner?

3. What methods would you use in carrying out Patricia Newman's teaching plan?

4. Assess the following factors that might affect Patricia Newman's learning.

Primary language

Memory

Vision

Barriers to learning

Secondary language

Hearing

Literacy level

5. Did you discover any cultural factors that might affect Patricia Newman's willingness to learn or the way you should plan teaching for her? Explain.

6. The nurse will expect which patient problem in the plan of care to address Patricia Newman's learning needs?

- Click on **Return to Nurses' Station** and then on **406**.
- Inside the patient's room, click on **Patient Care** and then on **Nurse-Client Interactions**.
- Select and view the video titled **1500: Discharge Planning**. (*Note:* Check the virtual clock to see whether enough time has elapsed. You can use the fast-forward feature to advance the time by 2-minute intervals if the video is not yet available. Then click again on **Patient Care** and **Nurse-Client Interactions** to refresh the screen.)
- After viewing the video, click on **Chart** and then on **406**. Select the **Patient Education** tab and read the education plan.

7. What seems to be missing from this plan, considering the video interaction you just viewed?

8. List eight areas of education that need to be addressed for Patricia Newman.

9. Consider the following areas of teaching in regard to Patricia Newman's care: diet management, disease condition, medication compliance, smoking cessation, activity, and self-care.

   a. Which of these teaching areas would be the first priority?

   b. Which would be the second priority?

10. Which of the following resources do you think would be helpful for your teaching plan? Select all that apply.

_____ Dietitian's help in planning meals

_____ Pictures of each medication

_____ Video on correct use of MDI

_____ Information and printed materials on community smoking cessation programs

_____ Drug inserts on her medications

_____ A chart for progress with progressive ambulation

_____ Booklet on emphysema and its treatment

_____ Statistics on death from smoking

_____ Chart and schedule for medication administration

_____ Demonstration of effective coughing

_____ Examples of high-protein snacks

_____ Pamphlet on proper MDI use

Exercise 2

Virtual Hospital Activity—Teaching Self-Injection

30 minutes

- Sign in to work at Pacific View Regional Hospital on the Medical-Surgical Floor for Period of Care 2. (*Note:* If you are already in the virtual hospital from a previous exercise, click on **Leave the Floor** and then on **Restart the Program** to get to the sign-in window.)
- From the Patient List, select Clarence Hughes (Room 404).
- Click on **Chart** and then on **404**. Click on the tab for **Nursing Admission** and read the assessment, noting factors that are pertinent to Clarence Hughes' learning.

1. Clarence Hughes states that he learns best by what methods?

2. How does Clarence Hughes describe his short- and long-term memory?

3. What problem does the patient indicate he has that will have an impact on teaching-learning sessions?

4. What would you do to help with this problem?

5. What other factor (specific to Clarence Hughes) needs to be considered when planning his teaching-learning sessions?

6. Once his pain is within tolerable limits, what teaching needs are important for Clarence Hughes?

7. Consider the events that have been taking place during Clarence Hughes' hospitalization. Identify the two greatest educational needs for him at this time.

_____   Prevention of osteoporosis

_____   Pain management

_____   Management/prevention of constipation

_____   Eating a balanced diet

8. Clarence Hughes will need to continue his enoxaparin injections at home. What methods could the nurse use to teach this skill? How would the nurse know that Clarence Hughes had learned to give his enoxaparin injections at home?

Exercise 3

Virtual Hospital Activity—Factors Affecting Learning

15 minutes

- Sign in to work at Pacific View Regional Hospital on the Medical-Surgical Floor for Period of Care 1. (*Note:* If you are already in the virtual hospital from a previous exercise, click on **Leave the Floor** and then on **Restart the Program** to get to the sign-in window.)
- From the Patient List, select Piya Jordan (Room 403).
- Click on **Go to Nurses' Station**.
- Click on **Chart** and then on **403**.
- Review the **Laboratory Reports** and the **Nursing Admission**.
- Click on **Physician's Notes** and review the notes.

1. Which of the following factors might interfere with Piya Jordan's ability to learn at the present time? Select all that apply.

_____   Fatigue

_____   Lack of family support

_____   NPO status

_____   Poor hearing

_____   Pain

_____   Nausea

_____   Tubes and drains

_____   Anemia

_____   Fear

_____   Confusion

_____   Inadequate oxygenation

2. Piya Jordan's best methods of learning are _____ and

_____.

3. What level of education does Piya Jordan have?

4. Piya Jordan was formerly employed as a(n) _____.

5. How might her former occupation be useful now?

6. If Piya Jordan's tumor turns out to be adenocarcinoma of the colon, she will need chemotherapy. How much support will her husband be able to provide?

7. What other support might be available to Piya Jordan?

8. What cultural factors should be taken into consideration when formulating a teaching plan for Piya Jordan?

Nursing Care of the Older Adult: Common Physical Care Issues

Reading Assignment: Promoting Healthy Adaptation to Aging (Chapter 13)
Safe Lifting, Moving, and Positioning Patients (Chapter 18)
Common Physical Care Problems of the Older Adult (Chapter 40)
Common Psychosocial Care Problems of Older Adults (Chapter 41)

Patients: William Jefferson, Skilled Nursing Floor, Room 501
Kathryn Doyle, Skilled Nursing Floor, Room 503

Objectives:

1. Identify interventions to assist the confused older adult patient.
2. Discuss age-related physiologic changes that predispose older adults to problems.
3. Examine factors related to polypharmacy.
4. Incorporate fall prevention measures into daily care.

Exercise 1

Virtual Hospital Activity—The Patient with Dementia

30 minutes

- Sign in to work at Pacific View Regional Hospital on the Skilled Nursing Floor for Period of Care 1. (*Note:* If you are already in the virtual hospital from a previous exercise, click on **Leave the Floor** and then on **Restart the Program** to get to the sign-in window.)
- From the Patient List, select William Jefferson (Room 501).
- Click on **Get Report** and review. Then click on **Go to Nurses' Station**.
- Click on **501** to visit William Jefferson. Read the Initial Observations.
- Click on **Chart** and then on **501**. Open the **History and Physical** and review.

1. What significant illnesses/disorders are discussed in William Jefferson's History and Physical?

2. According to the History and Physical, William Jefferson was diagnosed with Alzheimer's disease

    _____ years ago.

3. What stage of Alzheimer's disease is William Jefferson in?

4. Which of the following manifestations is associated with the late stage of Alzheimer's disease?
    a. Wandering
    b. Intermittent confusion
    c. Weight loss
    d. Incontinence

5. Which of the following are consistent with dementia-related memory problems, as opposed to normal age-related memory problems? Select all that apply.

    _____ Specific age of onset is easily established.

    _____ Patient seeks to conceal disability.

    _____ Patient actively uses memory aids such as notes.

    _____ Patient displays emotional lability.

    _____ Changes in abilities are common during the evening hours.

6. Indicate whether the following statement is true or false.

    _____ Anxiety can result in an older adult person displaying decreases in cognition.

7. Another term for sundowning is _____.

8. Indicate whether the following statement is true or false.

    _____ The terms *delirium* and *dementia* are interchangeable.

- Click on **Return to Room 501** and then click on **Patient Care**.
- Click on **Nurse-Client Interactions**.
- Select and view the video titled **0730: Intervention—Patient Safety**.
- Then select and watch the video titled **0740: The Confused Patient**. (*Note:* Check the virtual clock to see whether enough time has elapsed. You can use the fast-forward feature to advance the time by 2-minute intervals if the video is not yet available. Then click again on **Patient Care** and **Nurse-Client Interactions** to refresh the screen.)

9. What is the situation in the first (0730) interaction?

10. How does the second (0740) interaction demonstrate William Jefferson's confusion? What technique does the nurse use to handle the situation?

11. Indicate whether the following statement is true or false.

    _____ Given William Jefferson's confusion and attempts to ambulate on his own, restraints are indicated.

12. William Jefferson is concerned about the location of his dog. Based on your understanding, what impact do animals have on the confused older adult? Select all that apply.

    _____ Caring for animals is a source of stress for the confused older adult.

    _____ Animals provide a source of tactile stimulation.

    _____ Animal care provides a source of industry/purpose for the older adult.

    _____ Animals can fill the void of loneliness.

13. In planning care for William Jefferson, which of the following interventions is of the highest priority?
    a. Maintain adequate nutrition.
    b. Provide concise, direct instructions.
    c. Provide orientation to person, place, and time.
    d. Maintain physical well-being.

• Click on **Chart** and then on **501**. Select the **Nursing Admission** and read more about William Jefferson.

14. When caring for William Jefferson, the nurse may implement validation therapies. Which of the following is consistent with this therapeutic plan?
    a. Providing orientation to person, place, and time
    b. Encouraging him to keep a journal of his thoughts and feelings
    c. Encouraging him to reminisce about his life
    d. Using medication therapy to promote cognition

15. What social interaction does William Jefferson have when he is not in the hospital?

16. What impact does social interaction have on the older adult who is experiencing confusion?

Exercise 2

Writing Activity

15 minutes

Refer to a medical-surgical textbook if you need help answering the following questions.

1. How do decreased bladder tone and incomplete emptying predispose older adults to urinary tract infection?

2. What physiologic changes related to aging in males can contribute to the occurrence of the problems mentioned in question 1?

3. How does benign prostatic hypertrophy add to the problem of decreased bladder tone?

Exercise 3

Virtual Hospital Activity—Physical Problems of the Older Adult

30 minutes

Recall that William Jefferson was admitted with a urinary tract infection and sepsis. His diabetes and blood pressure were not controlled at the time of admission.

- Sign in to work at Pacific View Regional Hospital on the Skilled Nursing Floor for Period of Care 1. (*Note:* If you are already in the virtual hospital from a previous exercise, click on **Leave the Floor** and then on **Restart the Program** to get to the sign-in window.)
- From the Patient List, select William Jefferson (Room 501).
- Click on **Get Report** and read the report.
- Click on **Go to Nurses' Station**.

1. What is William Jefferson's most immediate need?
   a. Applying restraints to maintain safety
   b. Restricting fluids to prevent incontinence
   c. Preventing patient injury
   d. Administering medication for anxiety

William Jefferson developed sepsis, which in his case was a systemic inflammatory response to the infection. Sepsis can be fatal. It is important that the patient and his wife receive adequate teaching about prevention of future urinary tract infections. William Jefferson also has hypertension, diabetes, and osteoarthritis. Several medications have been prescribed for his various conditions.

• Click on **MAR** and select tab **501** for William Jefferson's records.

2. Below, list the regularly scheduled medication orders written for William Jefferson. For each medication, provide the action and explain why the patient is receiving it.

Medication Order	Action	Reason for Receiving

3. Rivastigmine has been prescribed for William Jefferson. Which of the following assessments is most important before administering his prescribed dosage?
   a. Intake and output
   b. Vital signs
   c. Level of cognition
   d. Reflexes
   e. Daily weight

4. Why is taking multiple medications such a problem for an older adult person?

5. The use of nonprescription drugs such as _____ or _____ can alter drug elimination from the body.

- Click on **Return to Nurses' Station**.
- Review William Jefferson's MAR and the Drug Guide as needed to answer the next question.

6. Discuss any age-related concerns with each of William Jefferson's ordered medications.

Exercise 4

Virtual Hospital Activity—Fall Prevention

15 minutes

- Sign in to work at Pacific View Regional Hospital on the Skilled Nursing Floor for Period of Care 1. (*Note:* If you are already in the virtual hospital from a previous exercise, click on **Leave the Floor** and then on **Restart the Program** to get to the sign-in window.)
- From the Patient List, select Kathryn Doyle (Room 503).
- Click on **Get Report** and read the report.
- Click on **Go to Nurses' Station**.
- Now click on **Chart** and then on **503**. Click on the tab for **History and Physical**.

Kathryn Doyle is in the Skilled Nursing Unit for rehabilitation after her hip surgery.

1. What medical conditions are listed in Kathryn Doyle's History and Physical?

- Click on **Return to Nurses' Station** and then on **503**.
- Click on **Clinical Alerts** and review the note.
- Click on **Patient Care** and then on **Nurse-Client Interactions**.
- Select and view the video titled **0730: Assessment—Biopsychosocial**. (*Note:* Check the virtual clock to see whether enough time has elapsed. You can use the fast-forward feature to advance the time by 2-minute intervals if the video is not yet available. Then click again on **Patient Care** and **Nurse-Client Interactions** to refresh the screen.)

2. What two factors did you discover that might contribute to Kathryn Doyle's risk for a fall? To what degree is she at risk for a fall?

3. Kathryn Doyle has a history of osteoporosis. This condition results in a loss of bone

    _____.

- Click on **Kardex** and review the activity orders for Kathryn Doyle.

4. What does the Kardex say about Kathryn Doyle's activity orders?

5. Kathryn Doyle has indicated a lack of interest in ambulation. What relationship exists between activity level and the development of osteoporosis?

- Click on **MAR** and then on tab **503** to review Kathryn Doyle's MAR.

6. Which of the following medications has been prescribed to treat Kathryn Doyle's osteoporosis?
    a. Calcium citrate
    b. Calcium carbonate

- Click on the **Drug Guide** and review the medication you identified in the previous question.

7. Which of the following side effects is most commonly associated with oral use of the medication identified in question 6?
    a. Nausea
    b. Mild constipation
    c. Flushing
    d. Diarrhea

8. When you help Kathryn Doyle to get up from the bed to sit in the chair, you should perform several actions in a particular sequence. Listed below are the actions you would need to take after positioning the chair next to the bed. Number these steps to show the order in which you would perform them. (*Hint:* Refer to Skill 18.4 in the textbook.)

Action	Order of Action
_____ Assist her to sit.	a. 1
_____ Put firm-soled slippers on her feet.	b. 2
_____ Place a transfer belt around her waist.	c. 3
_____ Ask her whether she is dizzy.	d. 4
_____ Sit her up on the side of the bed.	e. 5
_____ Allow a couple of minutes for her to dangle.	f. 6
_____ Allow a couple of minutes for her blood pressure to stabilize.	g. 7
	h. 8
_____ Help her to a standing position.	i. 9
_____ Tell her what you are going to do.	j. 10
_____ Lower the bed.	k. 11
_____ Assist her to the chair, gripping the transfer belt.	

• Click on **Return to Room 503** and then on **MAR**. Review Kathryn Doyle's MAR.

9. What medication is Kathryn Doyle receiving that could contribute to a fall? Why? (*Hint:* To check her medications for side effects, consult the Drug Guide [click on **Drug**] or use your pharmacology book or nursing drug handbook.)

Read about anemia in your medical-surgical textbook.

10. How can an anemic condition be a factor in a fall for an older adult person?

LESSON 7

Nursing Care of the Older Adult: Psychosocial Care

Reading Assignment: Growth and Development: Infancy Through Adolescence (Chapter 11)
Promoting Healthy Adaptation to Aging (Chapter 13)
Common Psychosocial Care Problems of Older Adults (Chapter 41)

Patients: Clarence Hughes, Medical-Surgical Floor, Room 404
William Jefferson, Skilled Nursing Floor, Room 501
Kathryn Doyle, Skilled Nursing Floor, Room 503

Objectives:

1. Identify the various types of elder abuse.
2. Determine factors that indicate an older adult person needs assistance.
3. Assess developmental level factors in older adults.
4. Describe factors that might indicate depression in older adults.

Exercise 1

Virtual Hospital Activity—Abuse, Depression, and Need for Assistance

30 minutes

- Sign in to work at Pacific View Regional Hospital on the Skilled Nursing Floor for Period of Care 3. (*Note:* If you are already in the virtual hospital from a previous exercise, click on **Leave the Floor** and then on **Restart the Program** to get to the sign-in window.)
- From the Patient List, select Kathryn Doyle (Room 503).
- Click on **Go to Nurses' Station**.
- Click on **Chart** and then on **503**.
- Click on the **Nurse's Notes** and review the note regarding the incident with a family member.
- Click on **Consultations** and **Nursing Admission** and review the data.

1. Depression is often overlooked in older adults. The physician has ordered a psychiatric nurse consult for Kathryn Doyle. What information have you found in her chart that might contribute to depression?

2. Identify the five types of abuse that may be experienced by older adults.

3. Older adults are most often abused by their _____ or their

   _____.

- Click on **Return to Nurses' Station** and then on **503** to visit Kathryn Doyle.
- Click on **Patient Care** and then on **Nurse-Client Interactions**.
- Select and view the video titled **1505: Assessment—Elder Abuse**. (*Note:* Check the virtual clock to see whether enough time has elapsed. You can use the fast-forward feature to advance the time by 2-minute intervals if the video is not yet available. Then click again on **Patient Care** and **Nurse-Client Interactions** to refresh the screen.)

4. Which of the following assessment findings for depression does Kathryn Doyle exhibit? Select all that apply. (*Hint:* Base your answers on the video interaction you just observed, as well as your review of the chart.)

_____ Fatigue

_____ Envy/criticism of others

_____ Appetite changes

_____ "Not feeling good"

_____ Sleep pattern changes

_____ Poor outlook on life

_____ Headaches

_____ Memory impairment

_____ Feelings of worthlessness/helplessness

5. The psychiatric nurse specialist suggests that Kathryn Doyle be started on a(n)

_____ of the _____ type.

6. When a patient is started on the type of medication identified in the previous questions, the primary

responsibility of the nurse is to _____.

7. Kathryn Doyle has not been taken to the dentist to have her dentures fixed for a very long time, and she

is having trouble eating. This could be considered as _____ on the part of her son.

8. Kathryn Doyle's son will not let her cook, clean, or manage her own money. She has indicated that she feels useless. These actions on the part of her son might be considered what type of abuse?

9. After a spouse dies, what signs would indicate that the surviving older adult spouse needs help and perhaps should not live alone? Select all that apply.

_____ Frequently unable to find the right words

_____ Forgetfulness

_____ Withdrawn from others

_____ Suspicious of others

_____ Confused about medications

_____ Watching a lot of TV

_____ Frequent falls

_____ Social isolation

_____ Not paying bills

10. What is the legal standard for nurses to report abuse?

Exercise 2

Virtual Hospital Activity—Therapeutic Communication and Medication

30 minutes

- Sign in to work at Pacific View Regional Hospital on the Skilled Nursing Floor for Period of Care 3. (*Note:* If you are already in the virtual hospital from a previous exercise, click on **Leave the Floor** and then on **Restart the Program** to get to the sign-in window.)
- From the Patient List, select William Jefferson (Room 501).
- Click on **Go to Nurses' Station**.
- Click on **MAR** and select tab **501**. Review William Jefferson's prescribed drugs.

  1. The physician has prescribed _____ for William Jefferson's Alzheimer's disease.

- Click on **Return to Nurses' Station** and then click on the **Drug** icon in the lower left corner of the screen. Scroll to the drug you identified in question 1 and read about it.

2. Below is a list of the possible side effects of the drug that has been prescribed for William Jefferson's Alzheimer's disease. Match each side effect with its degree of frequency.

Side Effect	Frequency of Side Effect
_____ Syncope	a. Frequent
_____ Nausea	b. Occasional
_____ Insomnia	c. Rare
_____ Tremor	
_____ Diarrhea	
_____ Anorexia	
_____ Hypertension	
_____ Anxiety	
_____ Headache	
_____ Confusion	

3. Does William Jefferson have other problems that this drug could exacerbate? If so, explain.

4. What would you teach William Jefferson and his wife about this drug?

- Click on **Return to Nurses' Station**.
- Click on **501** to visit William Jefferson.
- Click on **Patient Care** and perform a neurologic and mental status assessment by clicking first on **Head & Neck** (yellow buttons) and then on each of the subcategories (green buttons).
- After you have finished the assessment, click on **Nurse-Client Interactions**.
- Select and view the video titled **1525: Living with Alzheimer's**. (*Note:* Check the virtual clock to see whether enough time has elapsed. You can use the fast-forward feature to advance the time by 2-minute intervals if the video is not yet available. Then click again on **Patient Care** and **Nurse-Client Interactions** to refresh the screen.)

5. What is the first question the student nurse asks after sitting down?

6. The question you identified above is an example of what therapeutic communication technique?

7. William Jefferson says that when he can't remember, it makes him feel stupid. What does the student nurse say in response to this? What therapeutic technique is she using here?

8. What is the primary goal of psychosocial interventions for the confused or disoriented older adult?

9. What are the other principles of care for the cognitively impaired older adult?

Exercise 3

Virtual Hospital Activity—Developmental Tasks and Health Promotion

30 minutes

- Sign in to work at Pacific View Regional Hospital on the Medical-Surgical Floor for Period of Care 1. (*Note:* If you are already in the virtual hospital from a previous exercise, click on **Leave the Floor** and then on **Restart the Program** to get to the sign-in window.)
- From the Patient List, select Clarence Hughes (Room 404).
- Click on **Go to Nurses' Station**.
- Click on **Chart** and then on **404**.
- Click on the tab for **Nursing Admission** and review the data.

1. Clarence Hughes is _____ years old. He is in Erikson's stage of

   _____ and appears to be in _____ side of this stage.

2. What information tells you that Clarence Hughes is in the positive side of this developmental phase?

3. In contrast to Clarence Hughes, Kathryn Doyle is in the _____ side of this same developmental level. (*Hint:* Base your answer on what you learned about Kathryn Doyle in Exercise 1 of this lesson.)

4. What data from Exercise 1 support your answer to question 3?

5. Based on the data you have collected on Clarence Hughes, indicate how each of the following actions applies in his case.

Action		How It Applies
_____	Obtains a flu shot each year	a. Health-promoting for him
_____	Wears a seat belt when in the car	b. Risk to his health
_____	Obtains a prostate exam	c. Not done by him
_____	Smokes cigarettes	
_____	Drinks alcohol occasionally	
_____	Watches TV most of the time	
_____	Performs testicular self-exam	
_____	Keeps weight within a normal range	
_____	Takes a vitamin-mineral supplement daily	
_____	Uses medications for glaucoma regularly	

6. After his rehabilitation period, what health promotion behaviors would you recommend to Clarence Hughes?

7. What health promotion behaviors would you recommend for Kathryn Doyle?

Loss, Grief, and the Dying Patient

Reading Assignment: Cultural and Spiritual Aspects of Patient Care (Chapter 14)
Loss, Grief, and End-of-Life Care (Chapter 15)

Patient: Goro Oishi, Skilled Nursing Floor, Room 505

Objectives:

1. Describe the stages of grief and of dying, with their associated behaviors and feelings.
2. Discuss the concepts of hospice care.
3. List common signs of impending death.
4. Recognize the responsibilities of the nurse related to postmortem care.

Exercise 1

Virtual Hospital Activity—Advance Directives

30 minutes

- Sign in to work at Pacific View Regional Hospital on the Skilled Nursing Floor for Period of Care 1. (*Note:* If you are already in the virtual hospital from a previous exercise, click on **Leave the Floor** and then on **Restart the Program** to get to the sign-in window.)
- From the Patient List, select Goro Oishi (Room 505).
- Click on **Get Report** and read the report.
- Click on **Go to Nurses' Station**.
- Click on **Chart** and then on **505**.
- Click on and read the **History and Physical**, **Admissions**, and **Physician's Orders**.

1. Why was Goro Oishi admitted to the hospital, and what is his current status?

2. What plans for care are identified in the History and Physical?

3. Does Goro Oishi have an advance directive?

4. Indicate whether the following statement is true or false.

   _____ Goro Oishi's plan of care is a form of assisted suicide.

5. Which of the following are usually present in hospice care? Select all that apply.

   _____ Focus on symptom management

   _____ Focus on comfort care

   _____ Care for the family

   _____ Rigorous treatment of infection

   _____ Rigorous invasive measures to prolong life

   _____ Care in the hospital, home, or other facility

6. The type of care delivered within a hospice program is often termed

   _____.

7. Considering Goro Oishi's condition, his advance directive, and the principles of hospice/palliative care, which of the following nursing actions would be appropriate for him during this shift? Select all that apply.

   _____ Instill lubricating eye drops

   _____ Prepare to insert feeding tube

   _____ Assess IV site every 2 hours

   _____ Monitor oxygen saturation

   _____ Monitor urine output via Foley catheter

   _____ Medicate for nausea

   _____ Turn and reposition every 2 hours

   _____ Assess skin for pressure areas every 2 hours

   _____ Medicate for elevated temperature

_____ Get him up to the chair once during the shift

_____ Talk to him as care is provided

_____ Give him a bed bath

_____ Seek an order for treating constipation

_____ Provide urinary catheter care

• Click on **Return to Nurses' Station** and then on **505** to go to the patient's room.
• Inside the room, click on **Patient Care** and then on **Nurse-Client Interactions**.
• Select and view the video titled **0735: Assessment—Family**. (*Note:* Check the virtual clock to see whether enough time has elapsed. You can use the fast-forward feature to advance the time by 2-minute intervals if the video is not yet available. Then click again on **Patient Care** and **Nurse-Client Interactions** to refresh the screen.)

8. What do you think Mrs. Oishi means when she tells the nurse that she wishes her son would accept his father's wishes?

• Again, click on **Patient Care** and then on **Nurse-Client Interactions**.
• To complete the remaining questions in this exercise, you need to view two more nurse-client video interactions: **0745: Intervention—Clarification** and **0750: Family Conflict—Plan of Care**. (*Note:* Check the virtual clock to see whether enough time has elapsed. You can use the fast-forward feature to advance the time by 2-minute intervals if the video is not yet available. Then click again on **Patient Care** and **Nurse-Client Interactions** to refresh the screen.)

9. Match each Oishi family member with his or her present stage of grief.

Family Member	Stage of Grief
_____ Mrs. Oishi (patient's wife)	a. Denial
_____ Kiyoshi (patient's youngest son)	b. Anger
_____ Namishi (patient's oldest son)	c. Depression
	d. Acceptance

10. When planning care for Goro Oishi, the nurse must be aware of the potential impact of cultural norms. Which of the following beliefs is most often consistent with traditional Asian culture?
a. Individuals readily stand up to those in authority positions.
b. Health is viewed as a gift from God.
c. Individuals are reluctant to express their feelings to others.
d. Members of the church are considered to be like family.

11. An advance directive:
    a. states the patient's wishes in case of illness.
    b. spells out the patient's wishes for health care when the patient is unable to indicate his or her choice.
    c. legally appoints a person to carry out one's wishes.
    d. is aimed at prolonging life.

12. What are three advantages of having an advance directive in place?

13. Which of the following statements concerning the Physician Orders for Life-Sustaining Treatment form is correct? Select all that apply.

    _____   The form is available nationwide.

    _____   More than half of the states recognize the form.

    _____   The form is used most often for patients who have chronic progressive illnesses.

    _____   The form is widely recognized to assist families in making decisions for their incapacitated loved ones.

    _____   The form is initiated by a physician.

    _____   The form is initiated by the patient or durable power of attorney.

Exercise 2

Virtual Hospital Activity—Signs of Deterioration

30 minutes

In addition to an advance directive, a patient may have a signed durable power of attorney. Mrs. Oishi has the durable power of attorney for health care for Goro Oishi.

- Sign in to work at Pacific View Regional Hospital on the Skilled Nursing Floor for Period of Care 2. (*Note:* If you are already in the virtual hospital from a previous exercise, click on **Leave the Floor** and then on **Restart the Program** to get to the sign-in window.)
- From the Patient List, select Goro Oishi (Room 505).
- Click on **Get Report** and read the report.
- Click on **Go to Nurses' Station**.
- Click on **505** and then on **Take Vital Signs**.

1. Record Goro Oishi's current vital signs below.

   Blood pressure _____

   Oxygen saturation _____

   Temperature _____

   Heart rate _____

   Respiratory rate _____

- Click on and read the **Initial Observations** and the **Clinical Alerts**.
- Click on **EPR** and then on **Login**. Select **505** from the Patient drop-down menu and **Vital Signs** from the Category drop-down menu.
- Enter Goro Oishi's vital signs in the appropriate time column.
- Using the arrow at the bottom of the screen, scroll back to compare vital signs from previous times.

2. Complete the table below by entering Goro Oishi's vital signs from the EPR for the days and times specified.

Vital Sign	Mon 1545	Tues 0800	Wed 1130
Blood pressure			
Oxygen saturation			
Temperature			
Heart rate			
Respiratory rate			

3. What changes or trends do you see in the vital signs?

   Blood pressure: _____

   Oxygen saturation: _____

   Temperature: _____

   Heart rate: _____

   Respiratory rate: _____

4. Which of the following are physical signs of approaching death? Select all that apply.

_____ Temperature rises.

_____ Heart rate rises.

_____ Heart rate drops.

_____ Blood pressure rises.

_____ Blood pressure drops.

_____ Respirations become irregular.

_____ Extremities become mottled, cool, and dusky.

5. Considering the fact that Goro Oishi is comatose and unresponsive, it is impossible for the family to interact with him. What should the nurse caution the family to be careful about when in Goro Oishi's room?

- Click on **Exit EPR** to return to the patient's room.
- Click on **Patient Care** and then on **Nurse-Client Interactions**.
- Select and view the videos titled **1125: The Family Facing Death** and **1126: Supporting the Dying Patient**. (*Note:* Check the virtual clock to see whether enough time has elapsed. You can use the fast-forward feature to advance the time by 2-minute intervals if the video is not yet available. Then click again on **Patient Care** and **Nurse-Client Interactions** to refresh the screen.)

6. Does the younger son seem open to hearing any discussion of Goro Oishi's beliefs?

7. When working with the Oishi family members, what communication techniques can be used to assist them in dealing with the situation?

8. Indicate whether the following statement is true or false.

_____ The nurse's interaction with Goro Oishi's son provides him with information that enables him to accept his father's death.

- Click on **Patient Care** and then on **Nurse-Client Interactions**.
- Select and view the video titled **1128: The Medical Power of Attorney**. (*Note:* Check the virtual clock to see whether enough time has elapsed. You can use the fast-forward feature to advance the time by 2-minute intervals if the video is not yet available. Then click again on **Patient Care** and **Nurse-Client Interactions** to refresh the screen.)

9. Which of the following does Mrs. Oishi try to explain to her son? Select all that apply.

_____ She was chosen by her husband as his "agent" in case he reached the end of his life.

_____ She loves her husband and wants him to live.

_____ She wishes to respect her husband's wishes.

_____ She wishes to allow her husband to die with dignity.

_____ There is no way that her husband's condition will allow him to live.

10. Indicate whether the following statement is true or false.

_____ Goro Oishi's son's objection to the advance directive does not invalidate it.

Exercise 3

Virtual Hospital Activity—Signs of Impending Death

15 minutes

- Sign in to work at Pacific View Regional Hospital on the Skilled Nursing Floor for Period of Care 3. (*Note:* If you are already in the virtual hospital from a previous exercise, click on **Leave the Floor** and then on **Restart the Program** to get to the sign-in window.)
- From the Patient List, select Goro Oishi (Room 505).
- Click on **Get Report** and read the note.
- Click on **Go to Nurses' Station** and then on **505** to go to the patient's room.
- Read the Initial Observations.

1. A change noted in the Initial Observations that indicates Goro Oishi's kidneys have shut down is

_____ for the last 4 hours.

- Click on **Take Vital Signs**.

2. What are Goro Oishi's current vital signs?

Blood pressure_____

Oxygen saturation _____

Temperature _____

Heart rate _____

Respiratory rate _____

3. Compare these current vital signs with the ones you recorded earlier. What changes do you see in the vital signs now?

4. Cheyne-Stokes respirations may be noted as death approaches. Describe these respirations.

5. What causes the "death rattle" that may be heard near the end of life?

- Click on **Patient Care** and then on **Nurse-Client Interactions**.
- Select and view the video titled **1500: Patient Decline**.
- Next, select and view the video titled **1505: Meeting the Spiritual Needs**. (*Note:* Check the virtual clock to see whether enough time has elapsed. You can use the fast-forward feature to advance the time by 2-minute intervals if the video is not yet available. Then click again on **Patient Care** and **Nurse-Client Interactions** to refresh the screen.)

6. What change is happening to Goro Oishi?

7. The family requests that _____ be called.

8. Goro Oishi's vital signs have ceased, and the nurse has called the physician. Which of the following should the nurse also do now? Select all that apply.

_____ Ask the family members whether they wish to help prepare the body.

_____ Allow the family time alone with the patient.

_____ Remove tubes and cleanse the body.

_____ Prepare the body for the mortuary or coroner.

_____ Ask family members whether they want the nurse to stay with them while they spend this last time with the patient.

_____ Offer condolences.

Pain, Comfort, and Sleep

Reading Assignment: Cultural and Spiritual Aspects of Patient Care (Chapter 14)
Pain, Comfort, and Sleep (Chapter 31)
Complementary and Alternative Therapies (Chapter 32)

Patients: Clarence Hughes, Medical-Surgical Floor, Room 404
Pablo Rodriguez, Medical-Surgical Floor, Room 405
Kathryn Doyle, Skilled Nursing Floor, Room 503

Objectives:

1. Recall the parameters for assessment of pain.
2. Discuss the physiologic responses to pain.
3. Identify comfort measures to help relieve pain and promote rest.
4. Determine precautions for giving various analgesics.
5. Develop awareness of cultural and individual responses to pain.
6. Choose interventions to help the patient sleep and rest in the hospital.

Exercise 1

Virtual Hospital Activity—Pain Assessment

30 minutes

• Sign in to work at Pacific View Regional Hospital on the Medical-Surgical Floor for Period of Care 1. (*Note:* If you are already in the virtual hospital from a previous exercise, click on **Leave the Floor** and then on **Restart the Program** to get to the sign-in window.)
• From the Patient List, select Clarence Hughes (Room 404).
• Click on **Get Report** and read the report.
• Click on **Go to Nurses' Station** and then on **404**.
• Read the Initial Observations and click on **Clinical Alerts**.
• Click on **Take Vital Signs** and record them below.

1. What are Clarence Hughes' current vital signs?

   Blood pressure _____

   Oxygen saturation _____

   Temperature _____

   Heart rate _____

   Respiratory rate _____

   Pain rating _____

• Click on **EPR** and then on **Login**. Select **404** from the Patient drop-down menu and **Vital Signs** from the Category drop-down menu. Document the vital signs.

2. Are there any appreciable differences between Clarence Hughes' current vital signs and the previous vital signs?

3. Why is it important to measure other vital signs as part of the pain assessment?

4. When assessing pain, what four factors should be noted and documented?

5. Review Clarence Hughes' condition and complaints of pain. Which of the following pain types is he most likely experiencing?
   a. Chronic pain
   b. Nociceptive pain
   c. Neuropathic pain
   d. Phantom pain

• Click on **Exit EPR** and then on **MAR**. Select tab **404** for Clarence Hughes' MAR.
• Scroll through the MAR, noting the medication orders.

6. The medication ordered for Clarence Hughes' pain is _____.

• Click on **Return to Room 404.**
• Click on **Chart** and then **404**.
• Select the chart tab for **Expired MARs**.

7. According to the Expired MARs, how frequently has Clarence Hughes been receiving pain medication?

8. Clarence Hughes is at risk for what problem(s) while taking this medication?

9. What can be done to reduce the problem(s) identified in the preceding question?

- Click on **Return to Room 404**
- Click on **EPR** and then on **Login**. Select **404** from the Patient drop-down menu and **Gastrointestinal** from the Category drop-down menu.

10. Clarence Hughes had his last bowel movement _____.

11. The notes you have read indicate that the patient's knee and lower leg are swollen. How does this affect the pain level?

12. When Clarence Hughes' leg is not in the CPM machine, which of the following adjunctive measures might be used to decrease his pain? Select all that apply.

_____ Application of heat

_____ Application of cold

_____ Elevation of the leg and knee

_____ Distraction with a book, TV, or visitor

_____ Loud, lively music

_____ Favorite music softly played

_____ Imagery exercise

_____ Relaxation exercise

_____ Chiropractic manipulation

When a patient is admitted, it is always important to perform an assessment of spirituality, coping ability, and cultural preferences. What the assessment reveals should be woven into the plan of care.

- Click on **Exit EPR**. Now click on **Chart** and then on **404**.
- Select **Nursing Admission** and review this record.

13. Does Clarence Hughes have any particular spiritual beliefs or practices? If so, what are they?

14. Does Clarence Hughes indicate that he has good coping skills?

15. Does he have any special cultural practices?

Clarence Hughes doesn't have trouble sleeping at home, but in the hospital he finds uninterrupted sleep difficult. The physician has ordered medication to help him sleep.

- Click on **Return to Room 404** and then on **MAR**. Find the medication that is prescribed for sleep.

16. The physician has ordered _____ to help Clarence Hughes sleep. This drug should

   be given _____ before he wishes to fall sleep. This drug is classified as a(n)

   _____.

17. Which of the following side effects may be associated with the use of the medication you identified in the previous question? Select all that apply.

   _____ Nausea

   _____ Rebound lethargy

   _____ Euphoria

   _____ Weakness

   _____ Constipation

   _____ Anorexia

Exercise 2

Virtual Hospital Activity—Chronic Pain

15 minutes

- Sign in to work at Pacific View Regional Hospital on the Medical-Surgical Floor for Period of Care 1. (*Note:* If you are already in the virtual hospital from a previous exercise, click on **Leave the Floor** and then on **Restart the Program** to get to the sign-in window.)
- From the Patient List, select Pablo Rodriguez (Room 405).
- Click on **Get Report** and read the report.
- Click on **Go to Nurses' Station**.
- Click on **405** and then on **Take Vital Signs**.

1. Pablo Rodriguez has metastatic carcinoma of the lung and has been admitted with nausea, vomiting, dehydration, and poor pain control. What are his vital signs at this time?

   Blood pressure _____

   Oxygen saturation _____

   Temperature _____

   Heart rate _____

   Respiratory rate _____

   Pain rating _____

2. What type of pain do you think Pablo Rodriguez is experiencing?

- Click on **MAR** and note the medications Pablo Rodriguez is receiving.

3. What is ordered for pain management for Pablo Rodriguez?

4. Pablo Rodriguez is receiving _____ IV as an adjunctive medication to help control his pain.

- Click on **Return to Room 405** and then on the **Drug** icon in the lower left corner of the screen.
- Scroll to the medication you listed in question 4.

5. How do you think this medication helps decrease pain?

- Click on **Return to Room 405** and then click on **Chart**.
- Select the **Nursing Admission** and scroll to the sections on spiritual, cultural, and coping assessment.

6. What does Pablo Rodriguez say about his coping ability?

7. Where does he say his pain is located? How does he describe his pain?

8. Pablo Rodriguez's spiritual orientation is _____, and he feels that

_____.

9. If Pablo Rodriguez were able to take PO medications, what other type of adjunctive medications might help with his pain control?

10. Listed below are interventions used to help relieve pain. Match each specific intervention with its therapeutic type.

Intervention	Type of Measure or Therapy
_____ Reposition every hour	a. Adjunctive measure
_____ Keep lights low	b. Comfort measure
_____ Acupuncture	c. Complementary or alternative therapy
_____ Tricyclic antidepressants	
_____ Relaxation exercises	
_____ Imagery exercises	
_____ Change bed linens	
_____ Biofeedback	
_____ Soft music	
_____ Aromatherapy	

- Scroll to review the Rest and Activity portion of the Nursing Admission.
- Click on **Return to Room 405** and then on **MAR**.
- Review Pablo Rodriguez's MAR and note the medications ordered for him.

11. To help Pablo Rodriguez sleep, you would make sure that there are _____ available to help him get comfortable.

12. Is there a sleep medication ordered for Pablo Rodriguez?

Exercise 3

Virtual Hospital Activity—Factors That Influence Perception of Pain

20 minutes

- Sign in to work at Pacific View Regional Hospital on the Skilled Nursing Floor for Period of Care 2. (*Note:* If you are already in the virtual hospital from a previous exercise, click on **Leave the Floor** and then on **Restart the Program** to get to the sign-in window.)
- From the Patient List, select Kathryn Doyle (Room 503).
- Click on **Get Report** and read the report.
- Click on **Go to Nurses' Station**.
- Click on **EPR** and then on **Login**.
- Select **503** from the Patient drop-down menu and **Vital Signs** from the Category drop-down menu. Scroll backward in time through the vital signs findings.

1. Kathryn Doyle's pain has ranged from _____ to _____ on a scale of 1 to 10.

- Click on **Exit EPR** and then on **503**.
- Click on **Patient Care** and then on **Nurse-Client Interactions**.
- Select and view the video titled **1130: The Unexpected Event**. (*Note:* Check the virtual clock to see whether enough time has elapsed. You can use the fast-forward feature to advance the time by 2-minute intervals if the video is not yet available. Then click again on **Patient Care** and **Nurse-Client Interactions** to refresh the screen.)

2. What does Kathryn Doyle seem to be experiencing related to this interaction and the events that have occurred?

3. Which of the following factors do you think might make the perception of pain worse? Select all that apply.

_____ Pleasant visitors

_____ Fear

_____ Excessive noise

_____ Clean, quiet environment

_____ Anxiety

_____ Stress

_____ Inadequate sleep

_____ Attentive nurse

_____ Constipation

- Click on **MAR** and note the medications ordered for Kathryn Doyle.

4. What medication is ordered for pain for Kathryn Doyle?

5. Is there an adjunctive medication ordered that will help relieve her pain? If so, what?

6. The medication identified in question 4 tends to be constipating. What dietary recommendations would you make to help prevent Kathryn Doyle from experiencing constipation?

7. Kathryn Doyle has _____ ordered to help prevent constipation. (*Hint:* See the MAR.)

8. How does this medication work to help prevent constipation?

- Click on **EPR** and then on **Login**. Select **503** from the Patient drop-down menu and **Gastrointestinal** from the Category drop-down menu.

9. Kathryn Doyle had her last bowel movement _____ and _____ (is/is not) experiencing constipation.

10. Does Kathryn Doyle have anything ordered to help her sleep? If so, what? If not, why do you think nothing has been ordered?

- Click on **Exit EPR** and then on **Chart**.
- Select the chart for **503** and click on **Nursing Admission**. Scroll down to the section on Rest and Activity.

11. What does Kathryn Doyle do in preparation for sleep?

12. How might this activity interfere with her ability to sleep?

LESSON 10

Activity, Mobility, and Skin Care

Reading Assignment: Infection Prevention and Control in the Hospital and Home (Chapter 17)
Safe Lifting, Moving, and Positioning Patients (Chapter 18)
Assisting with Hygiene, Personal Care, Skin Care, and the Prevention of
Pressure Ulcers (Chapter 19)
Providing Wound Care and Treating Pressure Ulcers (Chapter 38)
Promoting Musculoskeletal Function (Chapter 39)

Patients: Harry George, Medical-Surgical Floor, Room 401
Clarence Hughes, Medical-Surgical Floor, Room 404
Patricia Newman, Medical-Surgical Floor, Room 406

Objectives:

1. Recognize areas of pressure that occur with different patient positions.
2. Recall risk factors that contribute to the formation of pressure ulcers.
3. Discuss the effects of immobility on the body's systems.
4. Assist patients to use devices that promote mobility.

Exercise 1

Virtual Hospital Activity—Complications of Immobility

30 minutes

- Sign in to work at Pacific View Regional Hospital on the Medical-Surgical Floor for Period of Care 2. (*Note:* If you are already in the virtual hospital from a previous exercise, click on **Leave the Floor** and then on **Restart the Program** to get to the sign-in window.)
- From the Patient List, select Clarence Hughes (Room 404).
- Click on **Get Report** and note pertinent information given in the report.
- Click on **Go to Nurses' Station** and then on **404**.
- Read the Initial Observations and the Clinical Alerts.
- Click on **Chart** and then on **404**. Select the **Physician's Orders**.

111

1. Clarence Hughes had a left total knee arthroplasty (replacement) on Monday. What are his current activity orders?

2. Clarence Hughes will be in a supine or semi-Fowler's position during the day in order to use the continuous passive motion (CPM) device; thus he will not be able to turn to his side. However, at night he may turn to the right side. Below, identify the pressure areas related to a supine position and those related to a side-lying position.

Pressure Area	**Position**
_____ Sacrum/coccyx	a. Supine position
_____ Occiput	b. Side-lying position
_____ Dorsal/thoracic area	
_____ Ischial tuberosity	
_____ Posterior knee	
_____ Malleolus	
_____ Lateral knee	
_____ Ilium	
_____ Trochanter	
_____ Shoulder	
_____ Elbow	
_____ Heel	
_____ Shoulder blade	

3. What are the purposes of using CPM after joint replacement?

4. When an area of redness is observed after turning a patient, what is the appropriate action?

   _____ Massage the area.

   _____ Reassess the area in 30 to 45 minutes.

   _____ Immediately check to see whether the area will blanch.

   _____ Apply a hot pack to the area.

5. As you are turning Clarence Hughes from a side-lying to a supine position during the night, you notice a reddened area on the right hip. The area does not blanch when you go back to check on it in an hour.

   You should chart that he has a stage _____ pressure ulcer.

6. If a stage 1 pressure ulcer has formed, which of the following should you do?
   a. Leave the area open to the air.
   b. Apply a hydrocolloid dressing.
   c. Apply a gauze dressing.
   d. Apply a transparent film dressing.

7. Clarence Hughes' new knee and its limited range of motion put him at risk for a fall. When he gets up to ambulate, you would teach him to do which of the following? Select all that apply.

   _____ Sit for a minute or two before standing.

   _____ Stand still until any dizziness passes before beginning to walk.

   _____ Wear firm-soled slippers.

   _____ Lean slightly forward while using the walker.

   _____ Maintain good, upright posture while ambulating.

   _____ Ambulate only when someone is holding on to him.

8. Because Clarence Hughes has had a knee joint replacement, he is at risk for neurovascular impairment. You should perform a neurovascular assessment on him every shift. Based on Clarence Hughes' age,

   the capillary refill in his toes should be _____.

9. To aid in the prevention of pressure ulcer formation, Clarence Hughes should be repositioned every

   _____ hours.

10. Describe how you would check sensation when performing your neurovascular assessment.

11. From the list below and on the next page, select the four effects of immobility on the musculoskeletal system.

    _____ Renal stones

    _____ Venous stasis

    _____ Decreased muscle mass and muscle tension

    _____ Negative nitrogen balance

    _____ Ischemia and necrosis of tissue

_____ Shortening of muscle

_____ Loss of calcium from bone matrix

_____ Decrease in bone weight

_____ Decreased independence

12. Because of the immobility caused by his surgical procedure, Clarence Hughes is at risk for the

    cardiovascular-respiratory complication called _____.

13. Clarence Hughes will be transported to the radiology department for a ventilation-perfusion lung scan. He will be transported by wheelchair. A major safety precaution when transferring a patient into or out of a wheelchair is to:
    a. place the chair to the left of the patient, who is seated on the bed.
    b. place the chair to the right of the patient, who is seated on the bed.
    c. move the leg extensions on the chair to the lowest position.
    d. check to see that the wheel locks are engaged.

Read in your textbook about the complication you identified in question 12.

• Click on **Return to Room 404**.
• Click on **Patient Care** and then on **Chest**.
• One at a time, click on each subcategory (green buttons) of the chest assessment.

14. Based on the change-of-shift report, the Initial Observations, the Clinical Alert, and your chest assessment, Clarence Hughes has shown which signs and symptoms consistent with complications of the respiratory system? Select all that apply.

    _____ Leaning forward

    _____ Diaphoresis

    _____ Coughing

    _____ Shortness of breath

    _____ Chest pain

    _____ Anxiety

    _____ Tachypnea

    _____ Production of frothy sputum

15. Identify respiratory-related complications that may result from immobility.

Exercise 2

Virtual Hospital Activity—Pressure Ulcer Risk and Infection

30 minutes

- Sign in to work at Pacific View Regional Hospital on the Medical-Surgical Floor for Period of Care 1. (*Note:* If you are already in the virtual hospital from a previous exercise, click on **Leave the Floor** and then on **Restart the Program** to get to the sign-in window.)
- From the Patient List, select Harry George (Room 401).
- Click on **Get Report** and review the report.
- Click on **Go to Nurses' Station** and then on **401**.
- Read the Initial Observations and Clinical Alerts notes.
- Click on **Chart** and then on **401**. Select the **Physician's Orders**.

1. What are the activity and positioning orders for Harry George?

2. When elevating Harry George's foot on pillows, you must be very careful to protect the

   _____ from pressure.

- Click on **History and Physical** and read through the form.

3. From the information in the History and Physical, what would you expect Harry George's nutritional status to be?

4. Which of the following factors cause a patient to be at greater risk for a pressure ulcer? Select all that apply.

   _____ Continued diaphoresis

   _____ Obesity

   _____ Weight loss

   _____ Incontinence

   _____ Bed rest

   _____ Dehydration

   _____ Confusion

   _____ Edema

   _____ Poor nutrition

5. Considering the data you have obtained, how many risk factors does Harry George have for developing a pressure ulcer? What are they?

- Click on **Physician's Notes** and determine what organism has caused the infection in Harry George's foot.

6. The organism causing the infection in Harry George's foot is

   _____.

- Click on **Return to Room 401** and then on **Patient Care**.
- Click on **Lower Extremities** and perform a focused assessment.

7. Below, record your findings from the focused assessment of Harry George's lower extremities.

Lower Extremity Assessment Areas	Harry George's Assessment Findings
Integumentary	
Musculoskeletal	
Vascular	
Neurologic	

- Click on **EPR** and then on **Login**.
- Select **401** from the Patient drop-down menu. Using the Category drop-down menu, select each appropriate category and document the assessment data you just obtained from Harry George.

8. The physician has ordered dressing changes for Harry George's foot. This procedure requires the use of standard precautions. Which of the following protective barrier items will be required to perform this dressing change? Select all that apply.

_____ Gloves

_____ Gown

_____ Mask

_____ Goggles

_____ Biohazard discard bag

_____ Private room

9. There are special criteria for transmission-based precautions in the hospital. Harry George's wound

would require _____ precautions.

10. When performing a dressing change for Harry George, you must adhere to principles of aseptic technique. Indicate the actions that adhere to aseptic principles while performing this dressing change. Select all that apply.

_____ Do not use dressings that have been opened but left in the room.

_____ Set up the sterile field above your waist height.

_____ Open sterile pack wrappers away from the body.

_____ Open the sterile glove pack on your sterile field.

_____ Place the discard bag at the back edge of the sterile field.

_____ Once gloved, keep your hands in sight.

Exercise 3

Virtual Hospital Activity—Physical Therapy to Increase Mobility and Endurance

15 minutes

- Sign in to work at Pacific View Regional Hospital on the Medical-Surgical Floor for Period of Care 4. (*Note:* If you are already in the virtual hospital from a previous exercise, click on **Leave the Floor** and then on **Restart the Program** to get to the sign-in window.)
- Click on **Chart** and then on **406**. Click on the **Consultations** tab and scroll to the PT/OT Consult. Read through the consultation notes. (*Remember:* You are not able to visit patients or administer medications during Period of Care 4. You are able to review patient records only.)

1. The plan states that Patricia Newman is to begin her pulmonary rehabilitation plan by walking

_____ minutes _____ times a day.

2. Patricia Newman is to walk _____ (independently/with assistance) for her activity plan.

3. What is the goal of Patricia Newman's physical therapy program?

4. Why is it important to evaluate Patricia Newman's weight-bearing ability? (*Hint:* Use critical thinking skills to answer this question.)

5. For which of the following activities does Patricia Newman require moderate assistance?

   _____ Bathing

   _____ Dressing

   _____ Toileting

   _____ Grooming

   _____ Eating

6. What might help Patricia Newman perform this daily activity task with less assistance?

7. The recommendations of the dietitian should be interwoven with the physical therapy plan. Why?

8. How might the exercise plan help to prevent further bouts of pneumonia? (*Hint:* Use critical thinking for this question.)

Vital Signs, Health Status Assessment, and Data Collection

Reading Assignment: Assessment, Nursing Diagnosis, and Planning (Chapter 5)
Measuring Vital Signs (Chapter 21)
Assessing Health Status (Chapter 22)

Patients: Pablo Rodriguez, Medical-Surgical Floor, Room 405
Patricia Newman, Medical-Surgical Floor, Room 406

Objectives:

1. Recognize abnormal vital signs.
2. Recognize factors that can affect vital signs.
3. Identify abnormal findings from the physical assessment.
4. Identify priority areas of assessment for specific patients.
5. Determine components needed to perform a focused assessment for identified actual or potential problems.

Exercise 1

Virtual Hospital Activity—Normal Versus Abnormal Vital Signs

45 minutes

Observing trends in vital signs often gives clues to patient problems.

- Sign in to work at Pacific View Regional Hospital on the Medical-Surgical Floor for Period of Care 3. (*Note:* If you are already in the virtual hospital from a previous exercise, click on **Leave the Floor** and then on **Restart the Program** to get to the sign-in window.)
- From the Patient List, select Pablo Rodriguez (Room 405).
- Click on **Get Report** and read the report.
- Click on **Go to Nurses' Station**.
- Click on **Chart** and then on **405**. Click on and review the **History and Physical**.
- Click on **Return to Nurses' Station** and then on **405** at the bottom of the screen.
- Click on **Take Vital Signs**. Record your findings in the top row of the table in question 2.
- Click on **EPR** and then on **Login**. Choose **405** from the Patient drop-down menu and **Vital Signs** from the Category drop-down menu.
- Use the blue arrows at the bottom of the screen to scroll to the previous vital sign recordings.

119

1. Why has Pablo Rodriguez been admitted to the hospital?

2. In the table below, enter Pablo Rodriguez's current vital signs and his earlier vital signs from the EPR. Based on these findings, begin to analyze the trend of each vital sign.

Day	Time	BP	SpO$_2$	T	HR	RR	Pain
Current findings							
Wed							
Wed							
Wed							

3. Review Pablo Rodriguez's blood pressure (current findings). When taking into account the impact of environmental factors and his alterations in comfort, which of the following best classifies his blood pressure?
   a. Normal
   b. Prehypertension
   c. Stage 1 hypertension
   d. Stage 2 hypertension

4. From your analysis of the vital sign trends, what do you think is causing the changes in Pablo Rodriguez's heart rate and respiration?

5. Which of the following factors or characteristics may result in an increase in pulse rate? Select all that apply.

   _____   Advancing age

   _____   Obesity

   _____   Sedatives

   _____   Anxiety

   _____   Blood loss

   _____   Physical activity

6. The normal adult range for temperature is _____. The normal heart rate

   range for an adult is _____. The normal range for respirations in the healthy adult is

   _____. The normal blood pressure for adults is _____.

7. Indicate whether the following statement is true or false.

   _____ The heart rate of an adult male is higher than that of an adult female of similar age.

8. Imagine you are applying the cuff of a manual sphygmomanometer to a patient's arm. From the list
   below, choose the appropriate steps for this procedure and number them in the correct order (from 1 to
   4). If a step is incorrect (does not apply to the sequence), choose "e."

Step	**Order of Steps**
_____ Place the cuff $\frac{1}{2}$ inch above the antecubital space.	a. 1
_____ Center the bladder over the brachial artery.	b. 2
_____ Verify that the cuff is $1\frac{1}{2}$ times the diameter of the patient's arm.	c. 3
_____ Wrap the cuff smoothly but securely around the arm.	d. 4
_____ Place the cuff 1 to 2 inches above the antecubital space.	e. Not a correct step in the sequence!
_____ Obtain a cuff that is 21% larger than the patient's arm.	

9. You need to measure a patient's respirations. Why would it be a good idea to tell the patient you are
   measuring the pulse instead?

10. In the list below and on the next page, select all choices that correctly complete the following
    statement. Taking an oral temperature would be contraindicated in a patient who:

    _____ has been running a high temperature elevation.

    _____ has had previous seizures.

    _____ has just finished breakfast.

    _____ is 7 years old.

    _____ suffers from dementia.

    _____ finished a cold soft drink 15 minutes ago.

_____ is newly postoperative.

_____ is a teenager with a leg fracture.

_____ is 2½ years old.

11. A rectal temperature is:
    a. 1 degree higher than an oral temperature.
    b. 1 degree lower than an oral temperature.

Exercise 2

Virtual Hospital Activity—Assessment and Data Collection

30 minutes

- Sign in to work at Pacific View Regional Hospital on the Medical-Surgical Floor for Period of Care 3. (*Note:* If you are already in the virtual hospital from a previous exercise, click on **Leave the Floor** and then on **Restart the Program** to get to the sign-in window.)
- From the Patient List, select Pablo Rodriguez (Room 405).
- Click on **Go to Nurses' Station**.
- Click on **Chart** and then on **405**. Review the **History and Physical**.
- Click on **Return to Nurses' Station** and then on **405** at the bottom of the screen.
- Inside the room, click on **Patient Care** and then on **Physical Assessment**.
- Click on **Chest** and then on each subcategory (green buttons). Note your findings.
- Click on **Abdomen** and then on each subcategory (green buttons). Note your findings.

1. Below, record your findings from the focused assessment of Pablo Rodriguez.

Assessment Area	Findings
Chest	
Integumentary	
Cardiovascular	
Respiratory	
Musculoskeletal	
Abdomen	
Integumentary	
Musculoskeletal	
Gastrointestinal	

2. Which of the following classifications best describes the assessment of Pablo Rodriguez's radial pulse strength?
   a. 1+
   b. 2+
   c. 3+
   d. 4+

• Click on **Chart** and then on **405**.
• Select **Nurse's Notes** and read through the notes.

3. List indications of problems that should be considered when writing Pablo Rodriguez's care plan.

4. Which of the following would the LP/VN expect to note as patient problems, considering the data you have gathered from your physical assessment and the chart? Select all that apply.

_____ Airway obstruction

_____ Constipation

_____ Decreased gas exchange

_____ Acute and chronic pain

_____ Decreased adherence

_____ Nausea

_____ Anxiety

_____ Fear

_____ Abnormal oral mucous membranes

5. Write one expected outcome for each of the nursing diagnoses you chose in question 4.

Exercise 3

Virtual Hospital Activity—Data Collection

30 minutes

- Sign in to work at Pacific View Regional Hospital on the Medical-Surgical Floor for Period of Care 3. (*Note:* If you are already in the virtual hospital from a previous exercise, click on **Leave the Floor** and then on **Restart the Program** to get to the sign-in window.)
- From the Patient List, select Patricia Newman (Room 406).
- Click on **Get Report** and read the report.
- Click on **Go to Nurses' Station**.
- Click on **Chart** and then on **406**.
- Click on **Nursing Admission** and read the admission pages.

1. Why has Patricia Newman been admitted to the hospital?

2. What medications was Patricia Newman taking at home?

3. Patricia Newman says her religion is _____.

4. She states that she smokes _____ packs per day.

5. Indicate whether the following statement is true or false.

   _____ Patricia Newman practices "preventive health care" by obtaining immunizations, doing breast self-exams, and living a healthy lifestyle.

6. What does Patricia Newman indicate is her goal for this hospitalization?

7. Patricia Newman says her normal bowel pattern is _____.

8. What sleep aid does she say she uses?

9. Does she have any hearing or vision difficulties or impairments?

10. Describe Patricia Newman's family relationships.

Exercise 4

Virtual Hospital Activity—Assessment

15 minutes

- Sign in to work at Pacific View Regional Hospital on the Medical-Surgical Floor for Period of Care 3. (*Note:* If you are already in the virtual hospital from a previous exercise, click on **Leave the Floor** and then on **Restart the Program** to get to the sign-in window.)
- From the Patient List, select Patricia Newman (Room 406).
- Click on **Go to Nurses' Station**.
- Click on **406** to go to the patient's room.
- Click on **Take Vital Signs**.

1. What are Patricia Newman's current vital sign measurements?

   Blood pressure _____

   Oxygen saturation _____

   Temperature _____

   Heart rate _____

   Respiratory rate _____

   Pain rating _____

2. When planning interventions to reduce Patricia Newman's temperature, which of the following may be included? Select all that apply.

_____ Lower the environmental temperature.

_____ Restrict fluid intake.

_____ Provide a cold sponge bath.

_____ Increase rate of air circulation.

_____ Remove bed coverings.

3. By definition, pyrexia occurs when the body temperature reaches or exceeds _____.

4. How can Patricia Newman's blood pressure be best described?
   a. Normal
   b. Prehypertension
   c. Stage 1 hypertension
   d. Stage 2 hypertension

• Click on **EPR** and then on **Login**.
• Select **406** from the Patient drop-down menu and **Vital Signs** from the Category drop-down menu.
• Review the vital sign patterns.

5. Patricia Newman's temperature recordings can best be described as:
   a. constant.
   b. intermittent.
   c. remittent.
   d. relapsing.

• Click on **Exit EPR**.
• Click **Patient Care** and then on **Nurse-Client Interactions**.
• Select and view the video titled **1500: Discharge Planning**. (*Note:* Check the virtual clock to see whether enough time has elapsed. You can use the fast-forward feature to advance the time by 2-minute intervals if the video is not yet available. Then click again on **Patient Care** and **Nurse-Client Interactions** to refresh the screen.)

6. What concerns and problems did you discover from the interaction?

• Because Patricia Newman's main problems are respiratory, click on **Physical Assessment** and then on **Chest**. Choose each subcategory (green buttons) to perform your assessment.

7. Below, record your findings for Patricia Newman's chest assessment.

Integumentary

Cardiovascular

Breasts

Respiratory

Musculoskeletal

8. The LP/VN should expect to see which four patient problems that are priorities for Patricia Newman?

Diagnostic Testing and Specimen Collection

Reading Assignment: Diagnostic Tests and Specimen Collection (Chapter 24)

Patients: Harry George, Medical-Surgical Floor, Room 401
Piya Jordan, Medical-Surgical Floor, Room 403

Objectives:

1. Recognize abnormal laboratory values.
2. Provide pre- and posttest teaching.
3. Recall the proper patient preparation for various diagnostic tests.
4. Explain the purpose of various diagnostic tests.
5. Explain what to expect during various diagnostic tests.

Exercise 1

Virtual Hospital Activity—Exploring Laboratory Values

30 minutes

- Sign in to work at Pacific View Regional Hospital on the Medical-Surgical Floor for Period of Care 3. (*Note:* If you are already in the virtual hospital from a previous exercise, click on **Leave the Floor** and then on **Restart the Program** to get to the sign-in window.)
- From the Patient List, select Harry George (Room 401).
- Click on **Go to Nurses' Station** and then on **Chart**.
- Click on **401** for Harry George's chart; then select the **Physician's Orders**.

1. In the list below and on the next page, identify the laboratory and diagnostic tests ordered for Harry George during this hospitalization. Select all that apply.

_____ Blood culture

_____ Ventilation perfusion scan

_____ CBC

_____ Chem 20

_____ Pulmonary function tests

_____ Bone scan

_____ Arterial blood gas

_____ Amylase and lipase

_____ Culture and sensitivity of wound

_____ KUB

_____ Clotting studies

_____ Folic acid level

_____ Alcohol level

_____ Chest x-ray

2. Discuss the relationship between Harry George's erythrocyte sedimentation rate and his admitting diagnosis.

3. When a blood chemistry panel is ordered, there is a requirement that _____ be

   withheld for _____ hours.

• Click on the **Laboratory Reports** tab and scroll to the urinalysis results.

4. Below and on the next page, list the values for Harry George's urinalysis. Consider how these findings compare with normal values. Place an asterisk (*) after any finding that is not normal.

Color

Character

Specific gravity

Acetone, ketones

Glucose

Protein

Nitrite

Occult blood

pH

Micro cells

Erythrocytes

Leukocytes

Bacteria

5. Harry George's urine is described as turbid. What is the character of normal urine?

6. A wound culture was ordered for Harry George. Which of the following must the nurse do when obtaining a wound culture? (*Hint:* See Skill 24-5 in your textbook.)
   a. Cleanse the entire wound thoroughly.
   b. Insert the sterile swab into the area where drainage is occurring.
   c. Put on exam gloves before opening swab container.
   d. Swab at least two sites in the wound with one swab.

7. Harry George has a bone scan (radionuclide study) ordered for his left foot. Which of the following statements by the nurse are appropriate in the teaching process to prepare him for the scan? Select all that apply.

   _____ "You must be NPO for 8 hours prior to the scan."

   _____ "A radioactive substance will be injected into a vein."

   _____ "You will be isolated while the radioactive substance is in your body."

   _____ "There will be a delay before the scan while the radionuclide is absorbed by the bone."

   _____ "You will be asked to empty your bladder after the scan."

   _____ "You will be radioactive for 24 hours."

   _____ "You will not be radioactive or a danger to others in the vicinity."

- Still in the **Laboratory Reports** section of Harry George's chart, scroll back to find his Hematology results.

8. A complete blood count (CBC) is often performed either to determine the presence of an infection in the body or to track whether treatment is clearing up an infection. When evaluating the CBC for signs

   of infection, you would check the number of _____ and the number of

   _____.

   Harry George's CBC values are _____ (normal/abnormal).

- Scroll to the Chemistry section of the Laboratory Reports.

9. Harry George's glucose level is _____. The normal range for blood glucose is

   _____.

• Scroll through the Chemistry section of the Laboratory Reports to find the albumin results.

10. Albumin is one measure of nutritional status of the body. Harry George's albumin level was

     _____. The normal range for albumin is _____.

11. Harry George's platelet count is monitored for the ability to _____.

12. Harry George's wound culture has been shown to be growing _____.

• Click on **Return to Nurses' Station** and then on **MAR**. Choose tab **401** for Harry George's MAR.

13. The first medication listed on Harry George's MAR is _____. This is an antibiotic, and it has a narrow therapeutic range. Peak and trough levels are ordered to track the amount of drug in Harry George's bloodstream.

• Click on **Return to Nurses' Station**; then click on the **Drug** icon in the lower left corner.
• Use the scroll button to find gentamicin in the drug listings. Read the information and note the therapeutic range for the peak and trough drug levels.
• Click on **Return to Nurses' Station** and then on **Chart**. Click on **401** and then on **Laboratory Reports**. Scroll down to the Drug Monitoring section of the reports.

14. Harry George's peak gentamicin level is _____. The trough level is

     _____. Normal therapeutic peak range for gentamicin is _____,

     and normal therapeutic trough range is _____. Toxicity occurs at a peak level greater

     than _____.

Exercise 2

Virtual Hospital Activity—Diagnostic Tests and Other Laboratory Tests

45 minutes

• Sign in to work at Pacific View Regional Hospital on the Medical-Surgical Floor for Period of Care 3. (*Note:* If you are already in the virtual hospital from a previous exercise, click on **Leave the Floor** and then on **Restart the Program** to get to the sign-in window.)
• From the Patient List, select Piya Jordan (Room 403).
• Click on **Go to Nurses' Station** and then on **403**.
• Read the Initial Observations.
• Click on **Chart** and then on **403**. Click on **Physician's Orders**.
• Read the orders, noting the laboratory and diagnostic tests that were ordered for Piya Jordan.

Piya Jordan was admitted with abdominal pain, and her diagnostic workup included several tests.

1. Below, match each test name with its appropriate type of test. (*Note:* Some letters will be used more than once.)

Test Name

Type of Test

_____ CT abdomen

__C__ Urinalysis

__b__ Hemoglobin and hematocrit

__e / g__ KUB and upright

__A__ Chem 7

__6__ PT/INR

_____ Chest PA & Lat

_____ Digoxin level

_____ Liver function

_____ Blood type and crossmatch (T&C)

a. Blood chemistry

b. Blood hematology

c. Urine test

d. Computer enhanced x-ray

e. X-ray

f. Blood clotting study

g. Blood drug monitoring

h. Blood serology test

2. What does a computed tomography scan show?

3. A KUB is an ___x-rau___ that shows the ___Kidneys, ureters & bladder___.

• Click on the **Diagnostic Reports** and read through the reports.

4. On the report of the CT of the abdomen, what was the impression of the radiologist?

5. The chest x-ray report for Piya Jordan was _____ (normal/abnormal).

• Click on the **Laboratory Reports** and review.

6. The current value for hemoglobin is _____.

   The current value for hematocrit is _____.

   The normal range for hemoglobin is _____.

   The normal range for hematocrit is _____.

   Piya Jordan is _____.

- Click on **Return to Room 403** and then on **MAR**. Select tab **403**. Note the digoxin order.
- Again, click on **Return to Room 403** and then on the **Drug** icon in the lower left corner. Scroll to find digoxin and read about this drug. Note the therapeutic range.

7. Piya Jordan has atrial fibrillation, which is being treated with digoxin. Digoxin has a narrow

   therapeutic range. The dose of digoxin ordered for Piya Jordan is _____ to be given

   daily.

- Once again, click on **Return to Room 403** and then on **Chart**.
- Choose **403** and click on **Laboratory Reports**.
- Scroll to the Chemistry section and find the potassium level.

8. Piya Jordan's potassium level is _____. The normal range for potassium is

   _____.

- Click on **Return to Room 403** and then on **MAR**. Select **403**.

9. How much potassium is Piya Jordan receiving?

- Click on **Return to Room 403**.
- Click on **Chart** and then on **403**.
- Select the **Laboratory Reports** and scroll down to the Special Tests section.

10. Piya Jordan's blood type is _____.

LESSON 13

Nutrition, Fluid, and Electrolytes

Reading Assignment: Fluid, Electrolyte, and Acid-Base Balance (Chapter 25)
Concepts of Basic Nutrition and Cultural Considerations (Chapter 26)
Nutritional Therapy and Assisted Feeding (Chapter 27)

Patients: Piya Jordan, Medical-Surgical Floor, Room 403
Pablo Rodriguez, Medical-Surgical Floor, Room 405

Objectives:

1. Identify nutritional components needed for healing.
2. Choose appropriate foods for basic therapeutic diets.
3. Perform teaching for various therapeutic/restricted diets.
4. Recognize abnormal electrolyte values.
5. Recognize risks of selected electrolyte imbalances.

Exercise 1

Virtual Hospital Activity—Individual Nutritional Needs

30 minutes

- Sign in to work at Pacific View Regional Hospital on the Medical-Surgical Floor for Period of Care 3. (*Note:* If you are already in the virtual hospital from a previous exercise, click on **Leave the Floor** and then on **Restart the Program** to get to the sign-in window.)
- From the Patient List, select Piya Jordan (Room 403).
- Click on **Go to Nurses' Station**.
- Click on **Chart** and then on **403**.
- Review the **History and Physical**.

1. In the previous lesson you determined that Piya Jordan is anemic. She is NPO at present, but when eating again, she will need dietary counseling. She has just had major surgery, and healing should be promoted. When healing from surgery or from a major wound, the body needs more

_____.

2. Vitamin B$_{12}$ can assist with hemoglobin synthesis. Which of the following menu selections will be beneficial to Piya Jordan once she resumes dietary intake?
   a. Citrus fruits
   b. Tomatoes
   c. Eggs
   d. Leafy vegetables

3. What is the impact on excessive protein intake in an individual who does not need it?

4. Piya Jordan weighs 114.4 lb (52 kg). Calculate the approximate daily protein needed to meet her normal daily needs.
   a. 42 g
   b. 65 g
   c. 143 g
   d. 150 g

5. Vitamin _____ plays a vital role in healing and should be increased in Piya Jordan's diet once she is eating.

6. Which of the following information is essential when assessing nutritional status? Select all that apply.

   _____ Age

   _____ Hours of sleep per night

   _____ Height

   _____ Occupation

   _____ Income level

   _____ Number of family members

   _____ Usual diet

   _____ Activity

   _____ Food preferences

   _____ General appearance

   _____ Weight gain or loss

   _____ Weight

   _____ Religion

• Click on and review the **Nursing Admission**.

7. Piya Jordan's weight is _____, and her height is _____.

8. What is Piya Jordan's BMI? Considering her height and weight, is her BMI within the acceptable range?

- Click on **Return to Nurses' Station** and then on **Kardex**.
- Select tab **403** and scroll to review the Fluid/Nutrition section of the Kardex.
- Next, review the Elimination section of the Kardex.

9. What is Piya Jordan's current diet order? What nutrition is she receiving?

10. Piya Jordan has a nasogastric tube in place. What are the potential functions of a nasogastric tube?

11. The physician has ordered that the nasogastric tube be connected to low intermittent suction. What is the underlying rationale of this order? (*Hint:* Refer to Skill 27-2 in your textbook.)

12. Earlier, you identified a vitamin that Piya Jordan needs to increase in her diet to aid in healing. She will also need additional iron to combat her anemia. Match each of the following foods with the nutrient(s) they will supply.

Food	Nutrient(s) Supplied
_____ Orange juice	a. Vitamin C
_____ Red meat	b. Iron
_____ Strawberries	c. Vitamin C and iron
_____ Legumes	
_____ Tomatoes	
_____ Green peppers	
_____ Potatoes	
_____ Whole grains	
_____ Green leafy vegetables	
_____ Fortified cereals	
_____ Grapefruit	

13. Piya Jordan will also need to have sufficient potassium in her diet. Because of her multiple nutritional needs, foods that supply two or more of her needed nutrients are especially valuable in her diet. Match the following foods with the nutrient(s) they supply.

Food	Nutrient(s) Supplied
_____ Bananas	a. Potassium
_____ Oranges	b. Potassium and vitamin C
_____ Broccoli	c. Potassium, vitamin C, and iron
_____ Carrots	d. Potassium and iron
_____ Potatoes	
_____ Meat	
_____ Legumes	
_____ Coffee	

14. After surgery, most patients begin eating with a(n) _____ diet and then progress until they are eating normally again.

Exercise 2

Virtual Hospital Activity—Fluid and Electrolyte Imbalance

30 minutes

- Sign in to work at Pacific View Regional Hospital on the Medical-Surgical Floor for Period of Care 3. (*Note:* If you are already in the virtual hospital from a previous exercise, click on **Leave the Floor** and then on **Restart the Program** to get to the sign-in window.)
- From the Patient List, select Pablo Rodriguez (Room 405).
- Click on **Get Report** and read the report.

1. What two factors mentioned in the shift report are likely to interfere with Pablo Rodriguez's nutritional intake?

2. When preparing to evaluate Pablo Rodriguez's skin turgor, which of the following sites may be used? Select all that apply.

_____ The abdomen

_____ The cheeks

_____ The thigh

_____ The forearm

_____ The palms of the hands

- Click on **Go to Nurses' Station** and then on **Chart**.
- Select **405** and click on **Emergency Department**. Read the entire section.

3. What two fluid and electrolyte problems did Pablo Rodriguez have when admitted to the Emergency Department?

4. List the sites of the body in which you can assess Pablo Rodriguez's skin turgor.

5. Which of the following are signs of dehydration? Select all that apply.

_____ Elevated temperature

_____ Elevated blood pressure

_____ Decreased urine output

_____ Increased heart rate

_____ Vomiting

_____ Postural hypotension

_____ Thick saliva

_____ Poor skin turgor

6. What signs of dehydration does Pablo Rodriguez exhibit in the Emergency Department?

- Click on **Laboratory Reports**. Scroll down to the Chemistry section and find the electrolyte values.

7. Record Pablo Rodriguez's electrolyte values for the days specified in the table below. Indicate whether each value is normal or abnormal.

Electrolyte	Tues	Normal or Abnormal?	Wed	Normal or Abnormal?
Sodium				
Potassium				
Calcium				
Phosphate				
Magnesium				

Read in your medical-surgical textbook about carcinoma of the lung. Note where this type of tumor is likely to metastasize.

- Click on the **History and Physical** and review.

8. A normal calcium level is _____ to _____.

9. What risk factor does Pablo Rodriguez have for hypercalcemia?

10. What two signs and symptoms of hypercalcemia does Pablo Rodriguez display?

11. Indicate whether the following statement is true or false.

    _____ Fluid intake should be limited when managing hypercalcemia.

12. If Pablo Rodriguez's calcium level continues to rise, he will be at risk for life-threatening

    _____.

13. How is Pablo Rodriguez's fluid imbalance treated in the Emergency Department?

It is important to treat Pablo Rodriguez's nausea and vomiting so that he can take in adequate nutrition and stabilize his fluid and electrolytes.

- Click on **Physician's Orders** and note the first medication ordered. Scroll down and note the drug ordered for nausea on Tuesday. Read all of the orders.
- Click on **Return to Nurses' Station** and then click on the **Drug** icon in the lower left corner. Read about these two drugs, which work differently.

14. The drug ordered for Pablo Rodriguez on Wednesday is _____.

    On Tuesday, the drug ordered for nausea was _____.

15. Why do you think Neutra-Phos was ordered for Pablo Rodriguez?

16. The diet the physician ordered for Pablo Rodriguez can be described as a(n)

    _____ diet.

17. Which of the following foods would be allowed on this diet? Select all that apply.

    _____ Whole milk

    _____ Lean meat

    _____ Cheese enchiladas

    _____ Baked fish

    _____ Ice cream

    _____ Butter

    _____ Margarine

    _____ Chili beans

    _____ Plain vegetables

Exercise 3

Virtual Hospital Activity—Calculating and Evaluating Intake and Output

15 minutes

- Sign in to work at Pacific View Regional Hospital on the Medical-Surgical Floor for Period of Care 3. (*Note:* If you are already in the virtual hospital from a previous exercise, click on **Leave the Floor** and then on **Restart the Program** to get to the sign-in window.)
- From the Patient List, select Pablo Rodriguez (Room 405).
- Click on **Go to Nurses' Station**.

- Click on **EPR** and then on **Login**.
- Choose **405** from the Patient drop-down menu **Intake and Output** from the Category drop-down menu.
- Scroll back to the Wednesday 0700 intake and output (I&O) results.

1. The shift intake for Pablo Rodriguez is _____ mL. His output was _____ mL.

2. Do you think that this indicates he is rehydrating? Explain.

- Using the scroll buttons, note the I&O amounts from 0700 to the current time.

3. Record the patient's I&O amounts below.

   Intake

   Output

4. Is there still a positive intake balance, indicating rehydration?

5. How many hours ago did Pablo Rodriguez last experience vomiting (emesis)?

6. Which of the following items could you offer Pablo Rodriguez to help rehydrate him? Consider his ordered diet and his postnausea status. Select all that apply.

   _____ Popsicle

   _____ Soft-boiled egg

   _____ Nonfat milk

   _____ Juice (clear)

   _____ Bouillon

   _____ Milkshake

   _____ Soft drink

   _____ Gelatin

   _____ Sherbet

LESSON 14

Promoting Respiration and Oxygenation

Reading Assignment: Fluid, Electrolyte, and Acid-Base Balance (Chapter 25)
Assisting with Respiration and Oxygen Delivery (Chapter 28)

Patients: Jacquline Catanazaro, Medical-Surgical Floor, Room 402
Patricia Newman, Medical-Surgical Floor, Room 406

Objectives:

1. Recognize abnormalities in oxygen saturation and other vital signs that indicate a respiratory problem.
2. Analyze trends in respiratory data.
3. Identify signs of hypoxia.
4. Safely administer oxygen.
5. State the purpose of various respiratory drugs.
6. Assist the patient with respiratory treatments.

Exercise 1

Virtual Hospital Activity—Respiratory Assessment

30 minutes

- Sign in to work at Pacific View Regional Hospital on the Medical-Surgical Floor for Period of Care 1. (*Note:* If you are already in the virtual hospital from a previous exercise, click on **Leave the Floor** and then on **Restart the Program** to get to the sign-in window.)
- From the Patient List, select Jacquline Catanazaro (Room 402).
- Click on **Get Report** for Jacquline Catanazaro and read the report.
- Click on **Go to Nurses' Station**.
- Click on **Chart** and then on **402**.
- Click on and review the **History and Physical** and **Nursing Admission**.

1. What are Jacquline Catanazaro's medical diagnoses?

2. Which of the following risk factors for the development of respiratory illness are present for Jacquline Catanazaro? Select all that apply.

_____ Age

_____ History of travel

_____ Occupational exposures

_____ Smoking

_____ Family history

_____ Inactivity

_____ Mental illness

- Click on **Return to Nurses' Station**.
- Click on **402** to enter the patient's room.
- Read the Initial Observations and Clinical Alerts.
- Click on **Patient Care** and proceed with a brief, focused respiratory assessment. First, click on **Chest** and then select subcategories **Respiratory** and **Musculoskeletal** (green buttons).

3. Below, record your findings from Jacquline Catanazaro's chest assessment.

Chest Assessment Area	Jacquline Catanazaro's Findings
Respiratory	
Musculoskeletal	

4. Is Jacquline Catanazaro's oxygen saturation level within normal limits? (*Hint:* See Skill 28-1 in your textbook.)

5. The pulse oximeter is a reading of:
   a. the level of the blood's hematocrit level.
   b. the oxygen saturation of hemoglobin in the blood.
   c. the body's level of $PaCO_2$.
   d. the body's acid-base balance.

6. Which of the following are considered to be early and/or initial signs of hypoxia? Select all that apply.

_____ Changes in level of consciousness

_____ Bradycardia

_____ Anxiety

_____ Temperature elevation

_____ Increased respiratory rate

7. Jacquline Catanazaro has bilateral wheezes. Which of the following best describes wheezing?
   a. High-pitched, whistling sounds
   b. Deep, snore sounds
   c. Rough, rubbing sounds
   d. Moist, popping sounds

• Click on **Take Vital Signs** and note the respiratory rate.

8. Jacquline Catanazaro's respiratory rate is _____. The normal adult respiratory rate is _____.

• Click on **Patient Care** and then on **Nurse-Client Interactions**.
• Select and view the video titled **0730: Intervention—Airway**. (*Note:* Check the virtual clock to see whether enough time has elapsed. You can use the fast-forward feature to advance the time by 2-minute intervals if the video is not yet available. Then click again on **Patient Care** and **Nurse-Client Interactions** to refresh the screen.)

9. During the respiratory crisis being experienced by Jacquline Catanazaro, what is the priority nursing diagnosis?
   a. Reduced stamina
   b. Anxiety
   c. Reduced gas exchange
   d. Inadequate health maintenance

10. What does the nurse tell Jacquline Catanazaro is the current plan?

• Click on **Chart** and then on **402**. Select the **Laboratory Reports** tab. Scroll down to the Arterial Blood Gas section.

11. In the table below, record Jacquline Catanazaro's arterial blood gas (ABG) results for the times specified.

ABGs	Mon 1030	Wed 0730
PaO$_2$		
O$_2$ sat		
PaCO$_2$		
pH		

12. Based on the ABG values above, what is Jacquline Catanazaro's acid-base abnormality?

Exercise 2

Virtual Hospital Activity—Respiratory Treatments

15 minutes

- Sign in to work at Pacific View Regional Hospital on the Medical-Surgical Floor for Period of Care 1. (*Note:* If you are already in the virtual hospital from a previous exercise, click on **Leave the Floor** and then on **Restart the Program** to get to the sign-in window.)
- From the Patient List, select Jacquline Catanazaro (Room 402).
- Click on **Get Report** for Jacquline Catanazaro and read the report.
- Click on **Go to Nurses' Station** and then on **Chart**.
- Select **402**. Click on **Physician's Orders** and read the most current orders.

1. What is the purpose of the nebulizer treatment that is ordered for Jacquline Catanazaro? What medication is ordered?

2. The medication referenced in the above question is classified as a(n) _____.

- Click on **Return to Nurses' Station**. Then click on the **Drug** icon in the lower left corner. Scroll to the drug ordered for the nebulizer treatment and read about it.

3. The normal adult dosage for a nebulizer treatment of this medication is _____ mg.

4. This drug has many side effects. Which problems that Jacquline Catanazaro is already displaying might be exacerbated by this drug? Select all that apply.

_____ Stuffy head

_____ Chest tightness

_____ Nervousness

_____ Headache

_____ Tachypnea

_____ Restlessness

_____ Excess salivation

• Click on **Return to Nurses' Station** and then on **MAR**. Select tab **402** and find the three drugs Jacquline Catanazaro is to receive by inhaler (puffs or metered-dose inhaler [MDI]). Record these drugs in the left column of the table in question 5 below.

• Once again, click on **Return to Nurses' Station** and then on the **Drug** icon. Find each of the three drugs you just listed in the table. As you read about each drug, record its purpose in the right column of the table.

5. In the table below, identify the three drugs Jacquline Catanazaro is to receive by inhaler. List the purpose of each of these drugs as well.

Inhaler Medication   **Purpose**

• You should have noticed in the MAR that Jacquline Catanazaro is also receiving prednisone. Read about this drug in the Drug Guide.

6. How do you think that prednisone helps a person with asthma?

7. When administering beclomethasone to Jacquline Catanazaro, which of the following instructions should be included? Select all that apply.

_____ Wait at least 2 minutes between inhalations.

_____ Rinse your mouth to reduce dryness and hoarseness.

_____ Shake the medication container well before use.

_____ Inhale and hold your breath as long as possible before exhaling.

Exercise 3

Virtual Hospital Activity—Oxygen Therapy

30 minutes

- Sign in to work at Pacific View Regional Hospital on the Medical-Surgical Floor for Period of Care 1. (*Note:* If you are already in the virtual hospital from a previous exercise, click on **Leave the Floor** and then on **Restart the Program** to get to the sign-in window.)
- From the Patient List, select Patricia Newman (Room 406).
- Click on **Get Report** and read the report.
- Click on **Go to Nurses' Station** and then on **Chart.**
- Click on the chart for **406** and then on **Physician's Orders**. Read the orders.

1. The physician has ordered oxygen at a rate of _____ by nasal cannula for

   Patricia Newman. The normal range for oxygen flow is _____.

2. An oxygen flow rate of 2 liters/min by nasal cannula provides the patient with _____% oxygen.

3. Although Patricia Newman's oxygen saturation is only 88%, the nurse does not increase the flow. Why is it unwise to increase the flow for this patient? (*Hint:* See the History and Physical to read about any long-standing disorders she has.)

4. Which of the following nursing actions are appropriate when a patient has oxygen ordered by nasal cannula? Select all that apply.

_____ Check nares to see that they are unobstructed.

_____ Observe for excoriation on the nose.

_____ Humidification is required if the flow rate is greater than 2 L/min.

_____ Humidification is always required when an oxygen cannula is used.

_____ Cleanse the nares each shift and check for signs of irritation.

_____ The cannula may be removed to make eating meals easier.

_____ Check the oxygen flow rate each time the room is entered to be certain it is set properly.

_____ Check the back of the patient's ears and the earlobes for signs of irritation each shift.

5. When a patient has oxygen ordered, safety measures must be instituted. What two things must the nurse do when instituting oxygen therapy?

- Still in the chart, click on **Diagnostic Reports** and read the chest x-ray report.

6. What does the impression note on the chest x-ray report say?

7. All patients with a respiratory ailment must be watched for signs of hypoxia. Which of the following is frequently the earliest sign of hypoxia?
   a. Constant cough
   b. Stridor
   c. Substernal retractions
   d. Restlessness

8. Hypoxia and respiratory insufficiency cause different signs and symptoms, depending on how long the patient has been hypoxic. Match each stage of hypoxia with the signs or symptoms common during that period.

Sign or Symptom	Stage of Hypoxia
_____ Cyanosis	a. Early
_____ Anxiety	b. Late
_____ Tachypnea	c. Latest
_____ Drop in blood pressure	
_____ Confusion	
_____ Muscle retractions	
_____ Stridor	
_____ Sitting up to breathe	
_____ Dysrhythmia	

9. In a person with emphysema, ineffective coughing spasms may lead to _____

   of the alveoli and may precipitate _____ of the airways.

10. Patricia Newman has pneumonia and a productive cough. She must cough effectively in order to clear her lungs of secretions. What type of coughing would you institute with her?

LESSON 15

Promoting Urinary and Bowel Elimination

Reading Assignment: Promoting Urinary Elimination (Chapter 29)
Promoting Bowel Elimination (Chapter 30)

Patients: Harry George, Medical-Surgical Floor, Room 401
Piya Jordan, Medical-Surgical Floor, Room 403
Pablo Rodriguez, Medical-Surgical Floor, Room 405

Objectives:

1. Identify factors in patient scenarios that interfere with normal urination.
2. Adequately assess elimination status of patients.
3. Recognize abnormal laboratory values for urine tests.
4. Describe proper urinary catheter care.
5. Describe factors that influence bowel elimination for patients.
6. List specific factors that contribute to elimination problems in patients.

Exercise 1

Virtual Hospital Activity—Urinary Catheter Care

30 minutes

- Sign in to work at Pacific View Regional Hospital on the Medical-Surgical Floor for Period of Care 1. (*Note:* If you are already in the virtual hospital from a previous exercise, click on **Leave the Floor** and then on **Restart the Program** to get to the sign-in window.)
- From the Patient List, select Piya Jordan (Room 403).
- Click on **Get Report** and review.
- Click on **Go to Nurses' Station**.

Piya Jordan is recovering from a colectomy. She has a Foley catheter in place, and as her nurse, you will be providing appropriate urinary catheter care.

1. Each time you enter Piya Jordan's room, you should check her urinary status by doing which of the following? Select all that apply.

_____ Check the urine in the bag for cloudiness.

_____ Switch the collection bag to the opposite side of the bed.

_____ Verify that the patient is not lying on the catheter.

_____ Irrigate the catheter.

_____ Check the connecting tubing to see that it is hanging straight to the collection bag.

_____ Make certain that urine is flowing into the bag.

_____ Do not raise the collection bag higher than the level of the bladder.

Because Piya Jordan is spending most of her time in bed, and because she has an indwelling catheter, she is at risk for a urinary tract infection. In order to assess her urinary status postoperatively, you need to know her preoperative urinalysis results.

- Click on **Chart** and then on **403**. Select **Laboratory Reports**.
- Scroll to the urinalysis results and record these results in the table in question 2.

2. Record Piya Jordan's urinalysis results below. In the right column, mark any abnormal results with an X.

Test	Piya Jordan's Results	Abnormal? (X)
Color		
Clarity		
Glucose		
Bilirubin		
Ketones		
Specific gravity		
Blood (occult)		
pH		
Protein		
Nitrite		
Micro: WBC		
RBC		
Bacteria		

It appears that Piya Jordan had a urinary tract infection before surgery. She was also dehydrated from vomiting, which can affect the test results. There was no time to treat the infection before her surgery, so the physician has ordered another urinalysis today.

3. Piya Jordan's urine specific gravity is elevated. What is specific gravity? What conditions impact this level?

4. To obtain a urine specimen from a patient with an indwelling catheter, you would clamp the catheter

   _____ the aspiration port for at least _____ minutes before obtaining the specimen.

5. You should use a(n) _____-gauge sterile needle and syringe to obtain the urine specimen from the aspiration port.

6. Aspirate _____ mL of urine for the urine specimen.

7. Below are the steps for obtaining a urine specimen. Show the correct order of steps by numbering the list from 1 to 12 (1 being the first step, 12 being the last).

   Steps of the Procedure

   _____ Wash hands; don gloves.

   _____ Unclamp the catheter.

   _____ Label the sterile container.

   _____ Check the order.

   _____ Clamp off the catheter.

   _____ Empty the syringe into the sterile container.

   _____ Aspirate the urine from the catheter.

   _____ Swab the aspiration port with alcohol.

   _____ Insert the needle into the aspiration port.

   _____ Instruct the patient about the procedure.

   _____ Close the sterile container.

   _____ Remove gloves; wash hands.

8. Changes can occur in urine if it sits at room temperature for very long. If a urine specimen cannot be

   taken to the laboratory immediately, it should be _____. It is best to send the labeled specimen, packaged in a biohazard bag, to the laboratory immediately.

9. Piya Jordan is at risk for bladder infection for a variety of reasons. Her risk factors include which of the following? Select all that apply.

_____ Urinary stasis from bed rest and inactivity

_____ Bowel colectomy

_____ Dehydration from nausea and vomiting before surgery

_____ NPO status with intravenous fluid administration

_____ Presence of an indwelling catheter

_____ Obesity

_____ Decreased bladder tone and possible incomplete emptying due to age

10. What is the single most important nursing measure to prevent infection in the patient who has an indwelling catheter? (*Hint:* Use critical thinking for this question.)

11. What signs and symptoms would you look for that might tell you your patient is experiencing a bladder infection (cystitis)?

12. People who are prone to recurrent bladder infections should drink plenty of water (2500-3000 mL a day) and should void at least every _____ hours.

13. When caring for Piya Jordan, the nurse must know that the hourly urine output should be at least:
    a. 25 mL
    b. 30 mL
    c. 35 mL
    d. 45 mL

- Click on **Return to Nurses' Station.**
- Click on **EPR** and then on **Login.**
- Select **403** from the Patient drop-down menu and **Intake and Output** from the Category drop-down menu.
- Review the urinary elimination patterns for Piya Jordan.

14. Indicate whether the following statement is true or false.

    _____ Piya Jordan has a urinary output that, when averaged, meets the minimum hourly amount.

Exercise 2

Virtual Hospital Activity—Assisting with Bowel Elimination

30 minutes

- Sign in to work at Pacific View Regional Hospital on the Medical-Surgical Floor for Period of Care 1. (*Note:* If you are already in the virtual hospital from a previous exercise, click on **Leave the Floor** and then on **Restart the Program** to get to the sign-in window.)
- From the Patient List, select Pablo Rodriguez (Room 405).
- Click on **Get Report** and review the report.
- Click on **Go to Nurses' Station**.
- Click on **405** to visit Pablo Rodriguez.
- Read the Initial Observations.
- Click on **MAR** and click on tab **405** for Pablo Rodriguez's MAR.

1. What medication is Pablo Rodriguez receiving that can cause constipation?

2. Refer to the preceding question. What impact does the medication have on bowel elimination?
   a. Slows peristalsis
   b. Draws water from stool in the lower colon
   c. Reduces neurologic stimuli related to the urge to defecate
   d. Slows the digestive processes in the stomach

- Click on **Return to Room 405**.
- Click on **Patient Care** and perform an abdominal assessment on Pablo Rodriguez. Record your findings in the table in question 3.

3. Record your findings from Pablo Rodriguez's abdominal assessment below.

Abdominal Assessment	Pablo Rodriguez's Data
Integumentary	
Musculoskeletal	
Gastrointestinal	

- Click on **EPR** and then on **Login**.
- Choose **405** from the Patient drop-down menu. From the Category drop-down menu, select **Gastrointestinal**. Enter your findings from the abdominal assessment in the correct EPR columns using the symbols listed for each line.

4. When did Pablo Rodriguez have his last bowel movement? What were the characteristics of his stool?

5. Why do you think Pablo Rodriguez is at risk for constipation and fecal impaction?

6. The physician has ordered a mineral oil enema. You know that the mineral oil enema should be

   retained for at least _____ in order to be effective.

• Click on **Exit EPR** and then on **MAR**. (Be sure you are looking at the correct page for Pablo Rodriguez!) Note the medications on the MAR that are used to prevent or treat constipation. Click on the **Drug** icon in the lower left corner to look up any medications with which you are unfamiliar.

7. Below, list the medications from Pablo Rodriguez's MAR that treat or prevent constipation. For each medication, list the action and/or use.

Medication	Action/Use

8. If the physician orders a soap suds enema for Pablo Rodriguez, there are specific steps to be followed.

   a. How would you position Pablo Rodriguez to administer the enema?

b. During a soap suds enema, how should the container be positioned?

c. What is the rationale for running the solution into the patient's body slowly?

d. What should be the temperature of the solution?

Exercise 3

Virtual Hospital Activity—Measures to Prevent Constipation

30 minutes

- Sign in to work at Pacific View Regional Hospital on the Medical-Surgical Floor for Period of Care 2. (*Note:* If you are already in the virtual hospital from a previous exercise, click on **Leave the Floor** and then on **Restart the Program** to get to the sign-in window.)
- From the Patient List, select Harry George (Room 401).
- Click on **Get Report** and review the report.
- Click on **Go to Nurses' Station**.
- Click on **Kardex** and then on tab **401**. Check what type of activity is ordered for Harry George.
- Click on **Return to Nurses' Station** and then on **Chart**. Click on **401** and then on **Nurse's Notes**. Read about Harry George's food intake.
- Click on **Return to Nurses' Station** and then on **MAR**. Select tab **401** and note the medications Harry George is taking that could contribute to constipation. (*Hint:* What pain medication is he receiving?)

1. How has Harry George been eating? What factors in his eating pattern could contribute to constipation?

- Once again, click on **Return to Nurses' Station** and then on **Chart**. Select the **Expired MARs** and read through them.

2. It appears that Harry George is receiving the pain medication _____

_____ about every _____. He has had _____ doses since admission.
    (*Hint:* Remember to check today's MAR also.)

- Click on **Nursing Admission** and review the Elimination section.

3. Harry George's usual bowel pattern is to have a bowel movement _____.

- Click on **Return to Nurses' Station** and then on **EPR**. Select **401** from the Patient drop-down menu and **Gastrointestinal** from the Category drop-down menu. Use the arrows to scroll back to see when Harry George last had a bowel movement.

4. Harry George's last bowel movement was _____.

   He _____ (does/does not) appear to be constipated.

5. Often bisacodyl suppositories are ordered prn in case the patient becomes constipated. How does this suppository work?

6. In addition to bisacodyl, what is another type of rectal suppository used to promote a bowel movement?

7. Many actions can help prevent elimination problems. For each action listed below, indicate whether the action can help prevent constipation (mark with "a"), help prevent urinary tract infection (mark with "b"), or help prevent both problems (mark with "c").

Action	**Elimination Problem It Helps Prevent**
_____ Increase fluids to 2500-3000 mL per day	a. Constipation
_____ Increase fresh fruits and vegetables in the diet	b. Urinary tract infection
_____ Exercise every day	c. Constipation and urinary tract infection
_____ Cleanse the perineum from front to back	
_____ Increase vitamin C intake	
_____ Empty the bladder after intercourse	
_____ Pay attention to the urge to defecate	
_____ Use aid such as hot coffee, hot water, and lemon juice	
_____ Avoid citrus fruits and juices	
_____ Wear cotton underwear	

Preparation for Drug Administration

Reading Assignment: Pharmacology and Preparation for Drug Administration (Chapter 33)
Administering Oral, Topical, and Inhalant Medications (Chapter 34)

Patients: Harry George, Medical-Surgical Floor, Room 401
Jacquline Catanazaro, Medical-Surgical Floor, Room 402

Objectives:

1. Give the rationale for why a patient is receiving a particular drug.
2. Calculate drug dosages accurately.
3. Identify the nursing implications for drugs a patient is to receive.
4. Describe the correct steps for administration of medications.

Exercise 1

Virtual Hospital Activity—Medication Knowledge

30 minutes

- Sign in to work at Pacific View Regional Hospital on the Medical-Surgical Floor for Period of Care 1. (*Note:* If you are already in the virtual hospital from a previous exercise, click on **Leave the Floor** and then on **Restart the Program** to get to the sign-in window.)
- From the Patient List, select Jacquline Catanazaro (Room 402).
- Click on **Get Report** and read the report.
- Click on **Go to Nurses' Station**.
- Click on **Chart** and then on **402**. Select **History and Physical** and review.

1. According to the History and Physical, what diagnoses and/or problems does Jacquline Catanazaro have?

- Click on **Return to Nurses' Station**, and then on **MAR**. Select tab **402** and find the medications requested in question 2 below.
- Again, click on **Return to Nurses' Station**. To complete question 2, consult the Drug Guide by clicking on the **Drug** icon in the lower left corner of your screen.

2. In the left column below, list the oral and topical medications ordered on Jacquline Catanazaro's MAR. For each medication, provide the reason she is receiving it.

Medication   **Reason for Receiving Medication**

3. Match each medication Jacquline Catanazaro is receiving with its classification or mechanism of action. (*Note:* Not all classification or mechanism of action options will be used.)

Medication	**Classification or Mechanism of Action**
_____ Prednisone	a. Antipsychotic/antidepressant
_____ Amoxicillin	b. Nonsteroidal antiinflammatory
_____ Ziprasidone	c. Antipsychotic
_____ Ibuprofen	d. Antibiotic
_____ Albuterol	e. Corticosteroid/systemic
_____ Beclomethasone	f. Bronchodilator/antiasthmatic
_____ Ipratropium bromide	g. Adrenocorticosteroid/antiinflammatory
	h. Anticholinergic/bronchodilator

4. Number the following steps for medication administration in the correct order.

Medication Administration Step	**Order of Steps**
_____ Check that this is the correct date and time the medication is ordered.	a. Step 1
_____ Check each medication against the MAR, comparing drug name, dose, and route as you pull it from the patient's drawer, bin, or automatic dispenser machine.	b. Step 2
	c. Step 3
_____ Verify that today's date is before the expiration of each medication.	d. Step 4
_____ Wash your hands.	e. Step 5
	f. Step 6
_____ Perform a second check of the medication for right drug, dose, time, and route.	g. Step 7
_____ Initial the MAR for each dose of medication administered.	h. Step 8
	i. Step 9
_____ Go to the patient.	j. Step 10
_____ Open the medication.	k. Step 11
_____ Verify the patient's identification by checking his or her armband against the name and number on the MAR and asking the patient to state his or her name.	
_____ Recheck each medication against the MAR for the right drug, dose, route, and time.	
_____ Administer the medications.	

• Return to the listing in the Drug Guide for prednisone.

5. Prednisone acts by:
   a. preventing release of corticosteroid in the body.
   b. increasing the release of adrenocorticosteroid.
   c. preventing tissue response to the inflammatory process.
   d. increasing the cell-mediated immune response.

6. Because of this action, prednisone may mask _____.

7. Patients who are receiving prednisone may experience _____ as a side effect, which makes them feel fatigued.

8. A bone disorder that occurs with long-term prednisone use is _____.

9. When a patient is receiving prednisone, the nurse must do appropriate teaching. Which of the following points would you cover in a teaching plan? Select all that apply.

_____ A single daily dose should be taken before 9:00 a.m.

_____ Take it only on an empty stomach, an hour before a meal.

_____ Report any other signs of infection.

_____ It is okay to have an occasional glass of wine while taking prednisone.

_____ Caffeine intake should be limited.

_____ Report weight loss promptly.

_____ Mood swings are not uncommon.

_____ Do not stop taking the drug abruptly.

10. You will be teaching Jacquline Catanazaro how to properly use her metered-dose inhaler (MDI) of albuterol. The proper steps are listed below. Number these steps in the proper order.

Steps for Using MDI for Albuterol	Order of Steps
_____ Wait 1 minute between puffs when more than one puff is ordered.	a. Step 1
_____ Place the mouthpiece 1 to 2 inches in front of your mouth.	b. Step 2
_____ Sit or stand up to use the inhaler.	c. Step 3
_____ Press the canister down while inhaling.	d. Step 4
_____ Shake the canister several times before beginning.	e. Step 5
_____ Breathe out through your mouth, emptying the lungs.	f. Step 6
_____ Use a bronchodilator MDI before a steroid MDI.	g. Step 7

• Scroll to find amoxicillin in the Drug Guide.

11. Are there any drug interactions between amoxicillin and the other drugs Jacquline Catanazaro is taking? If so, what are they?

12. What are the common gastrointestinal side effects of amoxicillin?

13. For the dose of amoxicillin ordered to be given at 1500, what would you do to try to prevent the gastrointestinal side effects?

Exercise 2

Virtual Hospital Activity—More Medications

30 minutes

- Sign in to work at Pacific View Regional Hospital on the Medical-Surgical Floor for Period of Care 1. (*Note:* If you are already in the virtual hospital from a previous exercise, click on **Leave the Floor** and then on **Restart the Program** to get to the sign-in window.)
- From the Patient List, select Harry George (Room 401).
- Click on **Get Report** and read the report.
- Click on **Go to Nurses' Station**.
- Click on **401** to visit the patient's room.
- Inside the room, click on **Check Allergies**.
- Now click on **Chart** and then on **401**; select the tab for **History and Physical**. Read about Harry George.

   1. What are Harry George's diagnoses and/or problems?

- Click on **Return to Room 401** and then on the **MAR**; review Harry George's MAR.
- Click on the **Drug** icon and review as needed to answer the following questions.

   2. Does Harry George have any allergies to medication?

   3. A medication may have a variety of therapeutic effects. Harry George has thiamine 100 mg PO or IM ordered. Which of the following is the most likely rationale for this order in his case?
      a. Reduces anorexia
      b. Increases effectiveness of antibiotic therapy
      c. Promotes carbohydrate metabolism
      d. Reduces ketones in the urine

4. The normal adult dosage of thiamine is up to _____.

   The order for Harry George _____ (is/is not) within the normal dosage range.

5. Are there any criteria that indicate the thiamine should be given intramuscularly?

- Click on **Return to Room 401**.
- Click on the **Drug** icon and scroll to gentamicin. Read about this drug.

6. What is the toxic level for gentamicin?

7. There are many nursing implications for gentamicin. Which of the following actions are the most important? Select all that apply.

   _____ Monitor intake and output.

   _____ Administer the drug between meals.

   _____ Ask the patient about ringing in the ears or decreased hearing.

   _____ Administer the drug only with a meal.

   _____ Report nausea promptly.

   _____ Give IM injection quickly.

   _____ Do not give if patient is dehydrated.

   _____ Assess for skin rash.

   _____ Report diarrhea promptly.

8. Are there any drug interactions between gentamicin and the other drugs Harry George is receiving?

9. Harry George has trimethobenzamide HCl 250 mg (Tigan) PO ordered q6h prn for nausea and

   vomiting. Trimethobenzamide HCl is a(n) _____ class drug.

10. Harry George is also receiving chlordiazepoxide HCl, and hydromorphone. What is the potential interaction effect of these drugs with trimethobenzamide HCl?

11. Harry George has glyburide ordered to help treat his diabetes. What is the mechanism of action of this drug?

12. What type or class of drug is glyburide?

13. Glyburide begins working within _____ minutes.

14. The glyburide is listed on the MAR to be given at 0800. What would the nurse need to know before administering the drug at that time?

15. Below, list the PO and topical drugs that are ordered for Harry George. For each drug, provide its action or the reason for administration.

Medication   **Action or Reason for Administration**

16. The physician has prescribed lorazepam to manage Harry George's agitation. This medication can best be described as which of the following?
    a. Schedule I
    b. Schedule II
    c. Schedule III
    d. Schedule IV
    e. Schedule V

- Click on **Return to Room 401**.
- Click on **Chart** and then on **401**.
- Click on **Laboratory Reports** and review Harry George's test results.
- Click on **Return to Room 401** and then on **Nurses' Station**.
- In the Nurses' Station, click on **Lab Guide** and consult as needed to answer the following question.

17. Which of Harry George's laboratory results should the nurse monitor for adequate kidney function?

18. Based on your review of the Harry George's laboratory results, should the gentamicin be given?

LESSON 17

Oral Medication Administration

Reading Assignment: Pharmacology and Preparation for Drug Administration (Chapter 33)
Administering Oral, Topical, and Inhalant Medications (Chapter 34)

Patients: Harry George, Medical-Surgical Floor, Room 401
Clarence Hughes, Medical-Surgical Floor, Room 404

Objectives:

1. Safely administer oral medications.
2. Identify the nursing assessments necessary before administering a drug.
3. Know the potential side effects and adverse effects of the drugs being administered.
4. Identify any interactions between drugs being administered and other drugs the patient is taking.

Exercise 1

Virtual Hospital Activity—Administering PO Medications

45 minutes

- Sign in to work at Pacific View Regional Hospital on the Medical-Surgical Floor for Period of Care 1. (*Note:* If you are already in the virtual hospital from a previous exercise, click on **Leave the Floor** and then on **Restart the Program** to get to the sign-in window.)
- From the Patient List, select Harry George (Room 401).
- Click on **Get Report** and review.
- Click on **Go to Nurses' Station** and then on **401**.
- Click on **Patient Care** and then on **Medication Administration**.
- Prepare to give Harry George his 0800 PO medications. (*Hint:* First click on **MAR** and find his orders.)

  1. Which oral medications is Harry George scheduled to receive at 0800 according to his MAR?

2. Are there any assessments that you need to make before preparing and administering these medications? (*Hint:* Harry George is diabetic, so you might want to know his morning blood glucose determination. Click on **Return to Room 401** and then on **Chart**. Select the chart for **401** and click on **Nurse's Notes**.)

3. Which of the following system assessments should you make before giving the 0800 PO medications? Select all that apply.

_____ Chest

_____ Abdomen

_____ Head & Neck

_____ Upper Extremities

_____ Lower Extremities

_____ Back & Spine

- Click on **Return to Room 401**.
- Now click on **Medication Room** and prepare Harry George's 0800 medications.
- Click on **Unit Dosage** and then on drawer **401** to access Harry George's medications.
- Click to highlight the correct drug to be removed from the drawer.
- Verify the MAR order against the medication information on dosage and route on the unit dose label (shown on the right side of the screen).
- Click on **Put Medication on Tray**.
- After each medication has been moved to the tray, click on **Review Your Medications** and again verify the drug, dosage, and route compared against the MAR information. This is your second check of the medication after removing it from the drawer.
- After your review of each medication, click on **Close Drawer** in the lower right corner of the screen and then click on **View Medication Room**.
- Now click on **Preparation** or on the tray sitting on the counter on the left side of your screen. Verify the drug label with the order and click on **Prepare**. This activates the Preparation Wizard. Supply any requested information; then click on **Next**.
- Click on the correct patient's room number and name and then click on **Finish**.

4. Below, document the medications ordered for Harry George at 0800.

Medication Order	Route	To Be Administered by You?

5. Glyburide can increase the activity of oral _____.

6. Is Harry George receiving the above-mentioned drug?

- Click on **Return to Medication Room** and then on **401**.
- Inside the patient's room, click on **Check Armband** to correctly identify Harry George as the patient for whom your medications are intended.
- Now click on **Check Allergies** and review this information.
- Click on **Patient Care** and then on **Medication Administration**.
- Click on the down arrow next to **Select**.
- Click on **Administer**. Choose the correct route from the drop-down menu. Next, select the correct method.
- Once you are sure everything has been checked three times and that the medication meets the order criteria and the correct time, click on **Administer to Patient**. Document that you have given the drug by clicking on **Yes**. Repeat this process for each medication on your tray. Finally, click on **Finish**.

7. What, if any, allergy does Harry George have?

- Click on the **Drug** icon and consult as needed to answer the following questions.

8. Glyburide peaks in _____ hours and lasts _____ hours.

9. Why is it important that Harry George eat his meals when he is taking this medication?

10. A patient taking glyburide should be monitored for which signs and symptoms of hypoglycemia? Select all that apply. (*Hint:* Consult the Drug Guide as needed.)

_____ Blurred vision

_____ Thirst

_____ Shakiness or tremors

_____ Rapid respirations

_____ Headache

_____ Tachycardia

_____ Hunger

_____ Cool, clammy skin

_____ Nausea or vomiting

_____ Increased urination

- Click on **Leave the Floor** and then select **Look at Your Preceptor's Evaluation**. Click on **Medication Scorecard** to see how you did with the medication administration for Harry George.

Exercise 2

Virtual Hospital Activity—Administering More Medications

30 minutes

- Sign in to work at Pacific View Regional Hospital on the Medical-Surgical Floor for Period of Care 1. (*Note:* If you are already in the virtual hospital from a previous exercise, click on **Leave the Floor** and then on **Restart the Program** to get to the sign-in window.)
- From the Patient List, select Clarence Hughes (Room 404).
- Click on **Get Report** and review.
- Click on **Go to Nurses' Station**.
- Click on **MAR** and note the medications to be administered to Clarence Hughes at 0800. (*Hint:* You will need to record these orders in the table in question 2.)
- Click on **Return to Nurses' Station** and then on **404** to go to the patient's room.
- Click on **Clinical Alerts** and determine what assessments need to be made before you administer medications. (*Hint:* You will use this information to answer question 5.)

1. What is the first thing you should do before going to the Medication Room and pulling medications for patients from the drawers or bins?

2. Below, copy the orders for the oral 0800 medications, as well as any prn medications, to be given to Clarence Hughes.

Medication Order	Route	Classification of Medication

3. What specific elements does a valid medication order contain?

4. Based on your review of the Clinical Alerts, what assessments should you perform?

- Click on **Check Allergies**.

5. Does Clarence Hughes have any drug allergies?

6. Is the order on the MAR for oxycodone with acetaminophen a valid order? If not, what is missing?

7. What should you do before giving the oxycodone with acetaminophen?

8. When administering medications to Clarence Hughes, it is important to be aware of the findings of

_____ research, which indicates that differing groups may metabolize medications differently.

- Click on **Medication Room** at the bottom of the screen.
- Click on **Unit Dosage** and then on drawer **404**.
- Click on the first medication you wish to administer to Clarence Hughes at 0800. Verify the unit dose medication label with the order as you take it from the drawer, following the six rights.
- Click on **Put Medication on Tray**. Continue this process for each medication that you are going to administer.
- Click on **Close the Drawer** and then on **View Medication Room** in the lower right corner.
- Click on **Automated System** to obtain the controlled drug. Click on **Login**.
- Select **Clarence Hughes, 404**. Choose the correct drawer for the medication you want. (Assume the order is for the 5/325 dosage.) Click **Open Drawer**.
- Select the correct medication and click on **Put Medication on Tray**. Then click on **Close Drawer**.
- Click on **Review Your Medications**. Highlight each medication in turn and perform your second medication check with the drug order. Use the six rights!
- Click on **Return to Medication Room** and then on **View Medication Room**.

9. What do you need to do before you prepare the medications you have put on the tray?

- Click on **Preparation** or on the tray on the counter on the left side of the screen.
- Click on **Prepare** and then supply any information requested by the Preparation Wizard before clicking **Finish**. Continue this process for each medication.
- Click on **Return to Medication Room**.
- Click on **404** to return to Clarence Hughes' room.

10. You have just entered Clarence Hughes' room. What should you do at this point?

11. When and how do you perform your third check of the medications?

- Click on **Patient Care** and then on **Medication Administration**.
- Follow the steps in the Administration Wizard until you have administered all the medications you prepared. (*Hint:* If you need help with any of these steps, refer to the **Getting Started** section of this workbook.)

12. What do you need to do after you have administered all of the medications for this time period?

- Click on **Leave the Floor**.
- Click on **Look at Your Preceptor's Evaluation**. Click on **Medication Scorecard** and review the evaluation.

Administering Injections and Topical Medications

Reading Assignment: Administering Oral, Topical, and Inhalant Medications (Chapter 34)
Administering Intradermal, Subcutaneous, and Intramuscular Injections
(Chapter 35)

Patients: Harry George, Medical-Surgical Floor, Room 401
Clarence Hughes, Medical-Surgical Floor, Room 404
Patricia Newman, Medical-Surgical Floor, Room 406

Objectives:

1. Correctly administer subcutaneous injections.
2. Identify injection sites for intramuscular injections.
3. Correctly administer an intramuscular injection.
4. Safely administer ophthalmic medications.
5. Use correct technique when applying a medicated skin patch.

Exercise 1

Virtual Hospital Activity—Administering Insulin

30 minutes

- Sign in to work at Pacific View Regional Hospital on the Medical-Surgical Floor for Period of Care 1. (*Note:* If you are already in the virtual hospital from a previous exercise, click on **Leave the Floor** and then on **Restart the Program** to get to the sign-in window.)
- From the Patient List, select Harry George (Room 401).
- Click on **Get Report** and review the information.
- Click on **Go to Nurses' Station**.
- Click on **401** to visit Harry George. Let's assume that when you ask the patient how he is feeling, he tells you that he is a little nauseous.
- Click on **MAR** and consult the Drug Guide to see what medication is ordered that may help relieve the nausea.
- Click on **Return to Room 401** and visit Harry George to see whether he needs anything else before you prepare this medication.

1. Harry George's MAR indicates he is to receive thiamine 100 mg once a day. What is the maximum safe dose for an adult?

Harry George says he can probably take his thiamine with a sip of water this morning.

- Click on **Medication Room** and then on **Unit Dosage**. Choose the drawer for **401**.
- Click on the correct drug to be removed from the drawer.
- Verify the MAR order with the dosage and route information on the unit dosage label.
- Click on **Put Medication on Tray**.
- Perform your second check of the medication by clicking on **Review Your Medications**. Once again, verify the drug, dosage, and route—and that it is intended to be given at this time on this date.
- Click on **Return to Medication Room**, then on **Close Drawer**, and then on **View Medication Room**.

2. What size syringe and needle will you choose to give this injection to Harry George?

3. What must you do before beginning to prepare the medications?

- Click on **Preparation** or on the tray on the counter. Verify the drug label against the order and click on **Prepare**. Supply any information requested by the Preparation Wizard; then click **Next**.
- Click on the correct room number; then click on **Finish** and then on **Return to Medication Room**.
- Click on **401** to return to the patient's room.

4. What should you do when you enter Harry George's room before giving his injection?

5. What precautions should you take when administering this injection?

- Now click on **Patient Care** and then on **Medication Administration**.
- Click on the arrow next to **Select** and choose **Administer**. After the Administration Wizard appears, choose the route, method, and site from the drop-down menus.
- Click on **Administer the Medication** and answer **Yes** to the next question.

6. The other site into which you could inject the thiamine is the _____.

7. Harry George has already had his early morning insulin. You will be giving him insulin before lunch later today. Before giving this next dose of insulin, what would you need to do?

8. When drawing up the indicated amount of insulin, what safety precaution should you take?

9. When both regular and NPH insulin are ordered to be given together, you would draw up the

   _____ insulin first.

10. Regular insulin has its onset in _____, peaks in _____, and has a duration of

    _____.

11. What area is preferred for insulin injection?

Exercise 2

Virtual Hospital Activity—Heparin Administration and Ophthalmic Medication Administration

30 minutes

- Sign in to work at Pacific View Regional Hospital on the Medical-Surgical Floor for Period of Care 1. (*Note:* If you are already in the virtual hospital from a previous exercise, click on **Leave the Floor** and then on **Restart the Program** to get to the sign-in window.)
- From the Patient List, select Clarence Hughes (Room 404).
- Click on **Get Report** and review the information.
- Click on **Go to Nurses' Station**.
- Click on **MAR** and check for the enoxaparin injection that Clarence Hughes is to receive.

1. Complete the table below based on the MAR order for enoxaparin.

Drug Order	Classification	Action	Precautions

2. What is the most likely reason enoxaparin is ordered for Clarence Hughes?

3. Enoxaparin is usually given after knee replacement surgery for an average of

   _____.

4. If Clarence Hughes experienced bleeding problems, you would give the antidote for enoxaparin,

   which is _____.

5. When administering enoxaparin, which of the following would you do to provide Clarence Hughes
   with the dose ordered? Select all that apply.

   _____ Use any subcutaneous site.

   _____ Use the prefilled syringe of 0.3 mL.

   _____ Use a 5/8-inch needle at a 45-degree angle.

   _____ Use a 1/2-inch needle at a 90-degree angle.

   _____ Use a 2-mL syringe.

   _____ Use the abdominal area lateral and below the umbilicus.

   _____ Pull the tissue taut before introducing the needle.

   _____ Pinch up the tissue in a roll before introducing the needle.

   _____ Inject deep into the subcutaneous tissue.

   _____ Do not aspirate before injecting this medication.

   _____ Rub the area gently after injection to hasten absorption.

   _____ Wait at least 15 seconds after injecting before withdrawing the needle.

6. Which life span consideration of this drug is of concern to Clarence Hughes?

• Return to Clarence Hughes' MAR and note the ophthalmic solutions ordered for him. Read about these medications in the Drug Guide.

7. Timolol and pilocarpine are used for what disorder?

8. If Clarence Hughes does not use his eye drops, what could be the consequences?

9. If these are new medications for Clarence Hughes, what points of patient teaching should you cover?

Exercise 3

Virtual Hospital Activity—Transdermal Medication

15 minutes

• Sign in to work at Pacific View Regional Hospital on the Medical-Surgical Floor for Period of Care 1. (*Note:* If you are already in the virtual hospital from a previous exercise, click on **Leave the Floor** and then on **Restart the Program** to get to the sign-in window.)
• From the Patient List, select Patricia Newman (Room 406).
• Click on **Get Report** and review the information.
• Click on **Go to Nurses' Station**.
• Click on **MAR** and then on tab **406**. Note the transdermal patch ordered for Patricia Newman.

1. Below, list the information for the transdermal patch ordered for Patricia Newman.

Medication Order	Classification	Action/Reason for Administration

2. Was the transdermal skin patch applied on Tuesday? (*Hint:* Go to the chart and check the Expired MARs to see whether the drug was administered.)

3. What should you do with the information you discovered?

4. Where should a skin patch be placed on the body?

5. After application, the patch should be _____ for identification of when it was applied.

6. When applying a new transdermal patch, you should always _____

_____.

7. What is necessary to do to ensure that the transdermal patch will adhere properly?

Caring for Patients Receiving Intravenous Therapy

Reading Assignment: Administering Intravenous Solutions and Medications (Chapter 36)

Patients: Harry George, Medical-Surgical Floor, Room 401
Piya Jordan, Medical-Surgical Floor, Room 403

Objectives:

1. Follow safe practice in the administration of intravenous (IV) fluids.
2. Identify signs of IV infiltration.
3. List the signs and symptoms of complications of IV therapy.
4. Perform assessments essential for the patient receiving IV fluids.
5. Monitor patients for side effects of IV medications.

Exercise 1

Virtual Hospital Activity—Monitoring the Patient Receiving Intravenous Therapy

30 minutes

- Sign in to work at Pacific View Regional Hospital on the Medical-Surgical Floor for Period of Care 1. (*Note:* If you are already in the virtual hospital from a previous exercise, click on **Leave the Floor** and then on **Restart the Program** to get to the sign-in window.)
- From the Patient List, select Harry George (Room 401).
- Click on **Get Report** and read the report.
- Click on **Go to Nurses' Station** and then click on **Chart**.
- Click on the chart for **401**. Select the tab for **Physician's Orders** and note the solutions and medications Harry George is currently receiving intravenously.

1. Below, list the IV solutions and medications ordered for Harry George. For each medication, give the classification, as well as its action or the reason it is ordered.

Medication Order	Classification	Action/Reason for Administration

You should become familiar with the side effects and nursing implications for these drugs because you are caring for Harry George.

2. Name the three most important nursing implications for the benzodiazepine drugs.

- Still in the patient's chart, click on **Nurse's Notes**.

3. According to the Nurse's Notes, on Harry George's arrival to the Medical-Surgical Floor from the ED, what site was used for the IV insertion?

- Click on **Return to Nurses' Station**.
- Click on **EPR** and then on **Login**.
- Select **401** from the Patient drop-down menu and **Intake and Output** from the Category drop-down menu.
- Determine Harry George's total PO intake for the past 12 hours.

4. For what reasons does Harry George require IV fluids and IV medications? (*Hint:* Review the Nurse's Notes and Physician's Progress Notes in the patient's chart for indications for IV medications.)

5. What question(s) would you ask Harry George about his IV site?

6. If tubing that delivers 15 drops per mL is being used, the IV will be flowing at _____ drops per minute.

7. Match each fluid with its correct classification of tonicity.

IV Fluid	**Tonicity**
_____ 0.9% Saline	a. Hypotonic
_____ 0.45% Saline	b. Isotonic
_____ 5% Dextrose in water	c. Hypertonic
_____ 10% Dextrose in water	
_____ 5% Dextrose in 0.9% saline	
_____ Ringer lactate	
_____ 5% Dextrose in Ringer lactate	

8. What is the purpose of administering an isotonic IV solution?

- Click on **Chart** and then on **401**. Click on **Nurse's Notes** and review.

9. As far as you can tell, when was Harry George's IV cannula inserted?

10. Is the IV cannula due to be changed today? Are there any indications that it should be changed? (*Hint:* Click on **Emergency Department** and read the ED nurse's notes.)

- Click on **Return to Room 401**.
- Click on **EPR** and then on **Login**. Select **401** from the Patient drop-down menu and **IV** from the Category drop-down menu. Highlight the data to see the pertinent abbreviations for interpretation of the documentation.

11. How often should Harry George's tubing be changed?
    a. Every 12 to 24 hours
    b. Every 24 hours
    c. Every 24 to 48 hours
    d. Every 72 hours

12. Identify complications that may result from IV therapy.

- When a patient is receiving IV fluid, the nurse should monitor the electrolyte values to determine whether the intravenous therapy is causing electrolyte imbalance.
- Click on **Exit EPR**.
- Click on **Chart** and then on **401**. Select **Laboratory Reports**.

13. Harry George's potassium level is _____. His sodium level is _____. His

    _____ level is above normal and most likely indicates a state of slight dehydration. The slightly elevated chloride level is consistent with the sodium level.

14. Which of the following laboratory reports would provide the best indication of whether the antibiotics Harry George is receiving are effective?
    a. Urinalysis
    b. Culture and sensitivity
    c. Complete blood cell count
    d. Gentamycin peak and trough levels
    e. Electrolyte panel

Exercise 2

Writing Activity—Complications of Intravenous Therapy

15 minutes

1. Match each sign or symptom with its related IV therapy complication. (*Note:* Some complications will have multiples signs or symptoms.)

Sign or Symptom	Complication of IV Therapy
_____ Coolness surrounding the IV site	a. Infiltration
_____ Redness at the IV site	b. Phlebitis
_____ Sudden drop in blood pressure with increase in pulse rate	c. Thrombophlebitis
_____ Redness of the vein used for IV therapy	d. Infection at site
_____ Red site with itching and rash	e. Air embolus
_____ Hardness along the vein used for IV therapy	f. Speed shock
_____ Fever, chills, general malaise	g. Infection
_____ Flushed face and severe headache	h. Circulatory overload
_____ Warmth at the IV site	i. Allergic reaction to IV medication
_____ IV flow sluggish with redness and tenderness at site	
_____ IV site hot, red, and painful	
_____ Elevated blood pressure, dyspnea, crackles in lungs	

2. What should you do if IV infiltration occurs?

3. If the IV flow has slowed considerably after the patient has been up for a sponge bath, what basic actions would you take before assuming that the cannula is clotted?

4. How often should you check on your patient to assess the IV site and flow rate when IV therapy is in progress?

5. You are monitoring your patient's IV. It is to run at 100 mL/hr. The tubing the hospital uses delivers 10 drops per mL. How many drops per minute should the IV deliver?
   a. 16 drops a minute
   b. 21 drops a minute
   c. 28 drops a minute
   d. 25 drops a minute

Exercise 3

Virtual Hospital Activity—Monitoring the Patient Receiving a Blood Transfusion

30 minutes

- Sign in to work at Pacific View Regional Hospital on the Medical-Surgical Floor for Period of Care 2. (*Note:* If you are already in the virtual hospital from a previous exercise, click on **Leave the Floor** and then on **Restart the Program** to get to the sign-in window.)
- From the Patient List, select Piya Jordan (Room 403).
- Click on **Get Report** and read the report.
- Click on **Go to Nurses' Station** and then on **Chart**.
- Click on **403** and select the **Physician's Notes**. Review to find out what blood product is planned for Piya Jordan.

1. The physician has planned to give Piya Jordan 2 units of _____.

2. Why is Piya Jordan receiving this blood transfusion? What laboratory parameters would you check before the blood is administered so that you will know later whether the transfusion was effective? (*Hint:* See the Laboratory Reports in her chart.)

3. In order for this blood product to be administered, Piya Jordan should have a(n)

   _____ IV cannula in place.

- Click on the **Nurse's Notes** and read the note for Wednesday at 0745.

4. Is the IV cannula that Piya Jordan has in place the correct size for the blood product transfusion?

5. Is there a valid consent signed by Piya Jordan for the blood transfusion?

6. Which of the following are pertinent guidelines when administering a blood transfusion? Select all that apply.

_____ Blood must be kept refrigerated until it is administered.

_____ Gloves must be used when discontinuing a blood product transfusion.

_____ Blood products are administered along with D_5W IV solution.

_____ Vital signs must be taken every hour while a blood product is infusing.

_____ Stay with the patient during the first 15 minutes of the infusion.

_____ The infusion should run at 2 mL/min for the first 15 minutes.

_____ Vital signs are taken every 30 minutes if they are stable after the first 15 minutes.

_____ Two nurses must verify the donor number, patient ID number, patient name, and ABO and Rh type on the blood bag, on the patient's blood armband, and on the slip accompanying the unit.

7. What is the average infusion time for a unit of packed red cells?
   a. 30 minutes
   b. 1 hour
   c. 2 hours
   d. 4 hours

8. Each patient must be carefully monitored for a transfusion reaction. Signs and symptoms of such a reaction include which of the following? Select all that apply.

_____ Chills

_____ Fever

_____ Abdominal pain

_____ Back pain

_____ Cramps in the legs

_____ Itching

_____ Shortness of breath

_____ Cough

9. What must be done immediately if a patient exhibits signs or symptoms of a transfusion reaction?

10. Most transfusion reactions occur within _____ of the infusion.

LESSON 20

Care of the Surgical Patient: Pre- and Intraoperative Care

Reading Assignment: Care of the Surgical Patient (Chapter 37)

Patients: Piya Jordan, Medical-Surgical Floor, Room 403
Clarence Hughes, Medical-Surgical Floor, Room 404

Objectives:

1. Identify preoperative procedures necessary for the patient scheduled for surgery.
2. List measures to be carried out for the patient to be readied for surgery.
3. Discuss care in the postanesthesia care unit (PACU).
4. Identify necessary elements of the PACU report to the floor.

Exercise 1

Virtual Hospital Activity—Preoperative Care

30 minutes

- Sign in to work at Pacific View Regional Hospital on the Medical-Surgical Floor for Period of Care 1. (*Note:* If you are already in the virtual hospital from a previous exercise, click on **Leave the Floor** and then on **Restart the Program** to get to the sign-in window.)
- From the Patient List, select Piya Jordan (Room 403).
- Click on **Get Report** and read the report.
- Click on **Go to Nurses' Station**.
- Click on **Chart** and then on **403**.
- Click on the **Surgical Reports** tab. Scroll to the Preoperative Patient Instruction Sheet.

1. Who is responsible for obtaining an informed surgical consent?
   a. The registered nurse
   b. The licensed practical nurse
   c. The anesthesiologist
   d. The primary care physician
   e. The surgeon
   f. The nursing supervisor

2. When providing information to the patient concerning a planned surgical procedure, which of the following must be included? Select all that apply.

_____ Risks of the planned operative surgery

_____ Alternative treatments available for the condition

_____ Possible complications during the postoperative period

_____ Cost of the surgical procedure

_____ Description of the procedure

3. When preparing to obtain the surgical consent from Piya Jordan, which of the following is the responsibility of the nurse?
   a. Explaining the procedure to Piya and her family
   b. Witnessing the signature of the patient
   c. Providing information concerning the risks and benefits of the procedure
   d. Ensuring the risks of the procedure have been explained to the patient

4. What instructions regarding hygiene were given to Piya Jordan in preparation for her surgery?

5. What were the instructions regarding eating or drinking?

6. According to the surgical admission sheet, Piya Jordan was scheduled for a(n)

   _____.

7. What does a colectomy involve? Why is it being done in Piya Jordan's case?

8. Which of the following risk factors for surgical complications apply to Piya Jordan? Select all that apply.

_____ Obesity

_____ Age

_____ Blood disorder

_____ Heart disease

_____ Respiratory disease

_____ Immune disorder

_____ Drug abuse

_____ Chronic pain

• Return to the **Surgical Reports** section of the chart. Scroll to the Surgery Procedures and Treatments form.

9. The preoperative sedation Piya Jordan received was _____.

Read in your pharmacology book or your nursing drug handbook about this medication.

10. Below, provide the requested information about the preoperative medication you identified in question 9.

Medication Order	Action	Onset and Duration

11. Which of the following are valid rationales for the administration of preoperative medications? Select all that apply.

_____ Preoperative medications are administered to reduce heart rate.

_____ Preoperative medications are administered to reduce nausea.

_____ Preoperative medications are administered to promote hydration during the surgical procedure.

_____ Preoperative medications are administered to enhance the effects of the anesthetic.

_____ Preoperative medications are administered to reduce the secretion of body fluids.

_____ Preoperative medications are administered to reduce mucus production.

12. Before administering preoperative medications, what must be checked or done?

13. When the nurse was teaching Piya Jordan about the use of the incentive spirometer preoperatively, what information should have been included?
    a. Inhale through the nose.
    b. Complete five full breaths for each session.
    c. Inhale completely and hold for at least 3 seconds.
    d. Exhale completely and hold for at least 10 seconds.

14. From the following list, identify the tubes and devices that Piya Jordan was told would be in place postoperatively. Select all that apply.

    _____   Abdominal binder

    _____   IV

    _____   NG tube

    _____   Foley catheter

    _____   Sequential compression devices (SCDs)

    _____   Abduction wedge

    _____   Patient analgesia controller

    _____   J-P suction device with drain

    _____   Traction apparatus

Exercise 2

Writing Activity—Intraoperative and Postanesthesia Care

15 minutes

1. Piya Jordan received _____ anesthesia.

2. The roles of the scrub nurse and the circulating nurse vary. Below, identify which functions each nurse would perform. (*Note:* If both nurses perform a function, choose c.)

Function	**Nurse**
_____ Sets up the instruments	a. Circulating nurse
_____ Conducts the "time out" surgical site identification	b. Scrub nurse
_____ Gowns and gloves the surgeon	c. Circulating nurse and scrub nurse
_____ Points out breaks in sterile technique	
_____ Counts sponges and instruments	
_____ Hands instruments to the operating team	
_____ Obtains needed fluids and medications	
_____ Takes charge of tissue specimens	
_____ Positions lights and stools	
_____ Assists with gowning and gloving	
_____ Checks function of each piece of equipment	
_____ Verifies that the electric cautery is properly grounded	
_____ Positions patient on the table and pads potential pressure areas	
_____ Communicates with those outside the operating room	

3. The _____ monitors the patient's vital signs during the operation.

4. When surgery is over, the patient is moved to the PACU and is positioned to

_____ and

_____.

5. In the PACU, the vital signs are measured and documented every _____ until

_____.

6. The Aldrete scoring system is often used to determine when the patient is ready for transfer back to the nursing unit. Which of the following areas are scored with this system. Select all that apply.

_____ Time in PACU

_____ Respiration

_____ Consciousness

_____ Gag reflex

_____ Skin color

_____ Circulation

_____ Activity

_____ Speech

7. Two important functions of the PACU nurse are to keep the patient _____ and to

reassure the patient that _____.

8. Because Piya Jordan has preexisting atrial fibrillation, the PACU nurse will monitor her closely. What assessments should the nurse perform related to this problem? (*Hint:* Use critical thinking for this question.)

Exercise 3

Virtual Hospital Activity—Another Surgery

30 minutes

- Sign in to work at Pacific View Regional Hospital on the Medical-Surgical Floor for Period of Care 1. (*Note:* If you are already in the virtual hospital from a previous exercise, click on **Leave the Floor** and then on **Restart the Program** to get to the sign-in window.)
- From the Patient List, select Clarence Hughes (Room 404).
- Click on **Get Report** and read the report.
- Click on **Go to Nurses' Station** and then on **404** to visit Clarence Hughes.
- Click on **Chart** and then on **404**. Click on **Surgical Reports**.

1. The surgical procedure that Clarence Hughes underwent was a(n) _____

_____.

2. Preoperatively, the nurse verified the disposition of Clarence Hughes' valuables. What does the preoperative form indicate as to the disposition of his valuables?

3. If Clarence Hughes had wanted to provide a preoperative autologous transfusion, it would need to have

   been completed _____ to _____ weeks before the scheduled surgery.

4. Because of the type of surgery Clarence Hughes had, he will not be able to exercise his foot and leg to the same extent that Piya Jordan is encouraged to do postoperatively; therefore he is at high risk for deep vein thrombosis. What would you encourage him to do with his lower left extremity?

5. What scheduled medications did the surgeon approve for Clarence Hughes to have in the immediate preoperative period?

6. Below, note the preoperative medication that Clarence Hughes received, along with the action, onset, and duration.

Preoperative Medication	Action	Onset and Duration

7. What procedures were performed on Clarence Hughes before the surgery was begun?

8. Clarence Hughes' surgery lasted _____.

9. What was tobramycin used for during this surgery?

10. What is in Clarence Hughes' history that makes it especially important for him to be diligent in using his incentive spirometer after surgery?

11. When teaching deep-breathing exercises to Clarence Hughes, the nurse should include what information?
    a. Deep-breathing exercises should begin the day after surgery.
    b. Deep-breathing exercises are best performed when sitting up with the back away from the mattress.
    c. Deep-breathing exercises should be preformed every 3 to 4 hours.
    d. Deep-breathing exercises should be performed with the patient sitting in low Fowler's position.

Care of the Surgical Patient: Postoperative Care

Reading Assignment: Nutritional Therapy and Assisted Feeding (Chapter 27)
Care of the Surgical Patient (Chapter 37)
Providing Wound Care and Treating Pressure Ulcers (Chapter 38)
Promoting Musculoskeletal Function (Chapter 39)

Patients: Piya Jordan, Medical-Surgical Floor, Room 403
Clarence Hughes, Medical-Surgical Floor, Room 404
Kathryn Doyle, Skilled Nursing Floor, Room 503

Objectives:

1. Discuss necessary elements of the postanesthesia care unit (PACU) report to the floor.
2. Identify assessments necessary for a patient returning to the nursing unit from surgery.
3. Prioritize care for the fresh postoperative patient.
4. Assist with convalescence and recovery after surgery.

Exercise 1

Virtual Hospital Activity—Postoperative Care After Knee Replacement

30 minutes

- Sign in to work at Pacific View Regional Hospital on the Medical-Surgical Floor for Period of Care 1. (*Note:* If you are already in the virtual hospital from a previous exercise, click on **Leave the Floor** and then on **Restart the Program** to get to the sign-in window.)
- From the Patient List, select Clarence Hughes (Room 404).
- Click on **Go to Nurses' Station** and then on **Chart**.
- Select the chart for **404** and click on **Physician's Orders**. Review the postoperative orders for Clarence Hughes.

1. What is the purpose of continuous passive motion (CPM) by machine after joint replacement surgery?

2. What would you do before placing Clarence Hughes' knee in the CPM machine?

3. What is the goal for the angle of flexion for Clarence Hughes today, the second postoperative day? Would you set the machine for this goal degree when beginning the procedure for the day?

4. How would you determine how well Clarence Hughes is tolerating the CPM machine?

5. Clarence Hughes is to ambulate twice a day. He will initially use a walker to do this. You know that the

   walker height is appropriate for him if his elbows are bent _____ degrees when his hands are on the handgrips and he is standing upright.

6. When checking the walker for safety, you would check to see that the

   _____ on the legs are intact.

- Click on **Return to Nurses' Station** and then on **404**.
- Inside the patient's room, click on **Patient Care** and then on **Chest**. From the list of assessment subcategories (green buttons), choose **Respiratory** and perform a respiratory assessment.

7. Clarence Hughes is at high risk of respiratory complications because he is a smoker. Record your findings from his respiratory assessment below.

- Now click on **EPR** and then on **Login**. Select **404** from the Patient drop-down menu and **Respiratory** from the Category drop-down menu.
- Document your assessment findings from above.
- Scroll back and review the previous respiratory findings review.

8. Has Clarence Hughes been using his incentive spirometer regularly?

9. Clarence Hughes is to use his incentive spirometer regularly. Check his orders and then decide which of the following teaching points you should go over with him. Select all that apply.

_____   Exhale through the nose.

_____   Inhale slowly and deeply.

_____   Hold the inhalation for 3 seconds.

_____   Use the spirometer for 20 breaths with each use.

_____   Breathe normally between each breath on the spirometer.

_____   Exhale into the spirometer forcefully.

_____   Use the spirometer ten times each hour while awake.

Exercise 2

Virtual Hospital Activity—Care of the Postoperative Patient

30 minutes

- Sign in to work at Pacific View Regional Hospital on the Medical-Surgical Floor for Period of Care 1. (*Note:* If you are already in the virtual hospital from a previous exercise, click on **Leave the Floor** and then on **Restart the Program** to get to the sign-in window.)
- From the Patient List, select Piya Jordan (Room 403).
- Click on **Go to Nurses' Station**.
- Click on **Chart** and then on **403**. Select **Physician's Orders** and review the postoperative orders.

1. After you receive a newly arrived postoperative patient and get report from the PACU nurse, what initial assessments would you make once the patient is settled in the unit?

2. What is the schedule for frequent vital sign measurements for a patient who has just returned from the operating room?

3. Piya Jordan needs to be repositioned every 2 hours. How can she be positioned after this surgery?

- Click on **Return to Nurses' Station** and then on **403**.
- Click on **Patient Care** and then on **Abdomen**.

4. Piya Jordan had an exploratory laparotomy and right hemicolectomy. For this reason, an abdominal assessment is of high priority. Assess all aspects of her abdominal area by clicking on each of the subcategories (green buttons). Then click on **Equipment** (to the right of the green buttons). Record your findings in the table below.

Additional Assessment Areas	Piya Jordan's Findings
Integumentary	
Musculoskeletal	
Gastrointestinal	
Equipment	

- Now click on **EPR** and then on **Login**. Select **403** from the Patient drop-down menu and **Gastrointestinal** from the Category drop-down menu.
- Next, choose **Wounds and Drains** from the Category drop-down menu.
- Document your findings from Piya Jordan's abdominal assessment.

5. What effect may Piya Jordan's age have on her wound healing?

6. Piya Jordan is presently in the _____ stage of wound healing, which lasts

   _____ days.

7. Piya Jordan has a(n) _____ wound drainage device.

8. What must be done after emptying the suction system in order to reactivate it?

9. Because Piya Jordan has had abdominal surgery, getting her to cough adequately will be difficult.
   Explain how you would prepare and assist her with coughing.

10. The physician has ordered sequential pneumatic compression devices for Piya Jordan. What is the
    purpose of these devices?

11. Piya Jordan's physician has ordered KCl be added to her IV fluids during the postoperative period.
    What assessment parameter must be considered when administering KCl to the patient?
    a. Respiratory rate
    b. Blood pressure
    c. Heart rate
    d. Temperature
    e. Intake
    f. Output

12. Which of the following will have the largest impact on determining when Piya Jordan will again be allowed to resume oral intake?
    a. Stabilization of vital signs
    b. Return of bowel sounds
    c. Quantity of drainage from Jackson-Pratt drain
    d. Decrease in drainage from nasogastric tube

Exercise 3

Virtual Hospital Activity—Surgical Recovery and Medication Administration

30 minutes

Kathryn Doyle is in the Skilled Nursing Unit, recovering from hip surgery.

- Sign in to work at Pacific View Regional Hospital on the Skilled Nursing Floor for Period of Care 1. (*Note:* If you are already in the virtual hospital from a previous exercise, click on **Leave the Floor** and then on **Restart the Program** to get to the sign-in window.)
- From the Patient List, select Kathryn Doyle (Room 503).
- Click on **Get Report** and read the report.
- Click on **Go to Nurses' Station** and then on **503**. Read the Initial Observations.

1. Kathryn Doyle has dry mucous membranes, which could indicate _____.

- Click on **Take Vital Signs**.

2. Record Kathryn Doyle's current vital signs below.

   Blood pressure _____

   Oxygen saturation _____

   Temperature _____

   Heart rate _____

   Respiratory rate _____

   Pain rating _____

- Click on **Patient Care** and perform a focused assessment on Kathryn Doyle, particularly looking for potential surgical complications.

3. What abnormalities did you find during the respiratory assessment for Kathryn Doyle?

4. What interventions can be implemented for Kathryn Doyle to improve her respiratory function?

5. Kathryn Doyle's Homans' sign was _____, and there is no evidence of the vascular

complication of _____.

- Click on **MAR** and see what medications are scheduled for Kathryn Doyle at 0800.

6. Below, list the medications you are to administer to Kathryn Doyle. For each medication, provide the classification and its action or the reason for giving it.

Medication Order	Classification	Action/Reason for Administration

- Click on **Medication Room** on the bottom of your screen and begin to prepare Kathryn Doyle's 0800 medications.
- Click on **Unit Dosage**. Select drawer **503**.
- Using the six rights, follow the onscreen steps to select the 0800 medications for Kathryn Doyle. For each selection, click on **Put Medication on Tray**.

7. In comparison with the orders, were there any problems with the medications that were in the drawer?

8. Based on your answer to question 7, how should you proceed?

- When all of the 0800 medications are on the tray, click on **Close Drawer**. Next, click on **Review Medications**, performing the second check for each dose ordered for 0800.
- Click on **Return to Medication Room** and then on **View Medication Room**.
- Click on **Preparation** or on the tray on the left side of your screen.
- For each medication, click on **Prepare** and provide the information requested by the Preparation Wizard.
- When all medications have been prepared, click on **Finish** and then on **Return to Medication Room**.
- Click on **503** to return to the patient's room. Click on **Patient Care** and then on **Medication Administration**.
- Administer each medication by clicking the down arrow next to **Select**, choosing **Administer**, and following the prompts.
- When you have finished the 0800 medication administration, click on **Leave the Floor** and then on **Look at Your Preceptor's Evaluation**. Click on **Medication Scorecard** to see how you did.

9. What three things should you have done before you rechecked and opened the medication unit dose packages?

Notes:

Notes:

Notes:

Notes:

Notes:

Notes:

Notes: